URBANIZATION AND SLUMS
Infectious Diseases in the Built Environment

PROCEEDINGS OF A WORKSHOP

V. Ayano Ogawa, Cecilia Mundaca Shah, and Anna Nicholson,
Rapporteurs

Forum on Microbial Threats

Board on Global Health

Health and Medicine Division

The National Academies of
SCIENCES · ENGINEERING · MEDICINE

THE NATIONAL ACADEMIES PRESS
Washington, DC
www.nap.edu

THE NATIONAL ACADEMIES PRESS   500 Fifth Street, NW   Washington, DC 20001

This activity was supported by contracts between the National Academy of Sciences and the U.S. Agency for International Development, U.S. Army Medical Research and Materiel Command (#10001249), U.S. Centers for Disease Control and Prevention (#10002642), U.S. Department of Homeland Security (#10003591), U.S. Department of Justice: Federal Bureau of Investigation, the National Institute of Allergy and Infectious Diseases/National Institutes of Health (#10003226), and the Uniformed Services University of the Health Sciences (#10003626), U.S. Food and Drug Administration (#10002125), and U.S. Department of Veterans Affairs (#10003353), and by the American Society for Microbiology, Infectious Diseases Society of America, Johnson & Johnson (#10003710), Merck & Co., Inc., Sanofi Pasteur, and Skoll Global Threats Fund (#1003664). Any opinions, findings, conclusions, or recommendations expressed in this publication do not necessarily reflect the views of any organization or agency that provided support for the project.

International Standard Book Number-13: 978-0-309-47439-9
International Standard Book Number-10: 0-309-47439-6
Digital Object Identifier: https://doi.org/10.17226/25070

Additional copies of this publication are available for sale from the National Academies Press, 500 Fifth Street, NW, Keck 360, Washington, DC 20001; (800) 624-6242 or (202) 334-3313; http://www.nap.edu.

Copyright 2018 by the National Academy of Sciences. All rights reserved.

Printed in the United States of America

Suggested citation: National Academies of Sciences, Engineering, and Medicine. 2018. *Urbanization and slums: Infectious diseases in the built environment: Proceedings of a workshop*. Washington, DC: The National Academies Press. doi: https://doi.org/10.17226/25070.

The National Academies of
SCIENCES · ENGINEERING · MEDICINE

The **National Academy of Sciences** was established in 1863 by an Act of Congress, signed by President Lincoln, as a private, nongovernmental institution to advise the nation on issues related to science and technology. Members are elected by their peers for outstanding contributions to research. Dr. Marcia McNutt is president.

The **National Academy of Engineering** was established in 1964 under the charter of the National Academy of Sciences to bring the practices of engineering to advising the nation. Members are elected by their peers for extraordinary contributions to engineering. Dr. C. D. Mote, Jr., is president.

The **National Academy of Medicine** (formerly the Institute of Medicine) was established in 1970 under the charter of the National Academy of Sciences to advise the nation on medical and health issues. Members are elected by their peers for distinguished contributions to medicine and health. Dr. Victor J. Dzau is president.

The three Academies work together as the **National Academies of Sciences, Engineering, and Medicine** to provide independent, objective analysis and advice to the nation and conduct other activities to solve complex problems and inform public policy decisions. The National Academies also encourage education and research, recognize outstanding contributions to knowledge, and increase public understanding in matters of science, engineering, and medicine.

Learn more about the National Academies of Sciences, Engineering, and Medicine at **www.nationalacademies.org**.

The National Academies of
SCIENCES • ENGINEERING • MEDICINE

Consensus Study Reports published by the National Academies of Sciences, Engineering, and Medicine document the evidence-based consensus on the study's statement of task by an authoring committee of experts. Reports typically include findings, conclusions, and recommendations based on information gathered by the committee and the committee's deliberations. Each report has been subjected to a rigorous and independent peer-review process and it represents the position of the National Academies on the statement of task.

Proceedings published by the National Academies of Sciences, Engineering, and Medicine chronicle the presentations and discussions at a workshop, symposium, or other event convened by the National Academies. The statements and opinions contained in proceedings are those of the participants and are not endorsed by other participants, the planning committee, or the National Academies.

For information about other products and activities of the National Academies, please visit www.nationalacademies.org/about/whatwedo.

PLANNING COMMITTEE ON URBANIZATION AND SLUMS: INFECTIOUS DISEASES IN THE BUILT ENVIRONMENT[1]

JAMES M. HUGHES (*Co-Chair*), Professor of Medicine and Public Health, Rollins School of Public Health, Emory University
MARY E. WILSON (*Co-Chair*), Clinical Professor of Epidemiology and Biostatistics, School of Medicine, University of California, San Francisco
JASON CORBURN, Professor of Public Health and of City and Regional Planning; Director, Institute of Urban and Regional Development, University of California, Berkeley
MARIA GLORIA DOMINGUEZ-BELLO, Associate Professor of Medicine, New York University School of Medicine
MARCOS A. ESPINAL, Director, Department of Communicable Diseases and Health Analysis, Pan American Health Organization
EVA HARRIS, Professor, Division of Infectious Disease and Vaccinology; Director, Center for Global Public Health, University of California, Berkeley
MARK T. HERNANDEZ, Professor of Environmental Engineering, University of Colorado Boulder
ALBERT ICKSANG KO, Professor and Chair, Department of Epidemiology of Microbial Diseases, Yale School of Public Health
ERIC MINTZ, Team Lead, Global Epidemiology, Waterborne Disease Prevention Branch, U.S. Centers for Disease Control and Prevention
THOMAS W. SCOTT, Distinguished Professor, Department of Entomology and Nematology, University of California, Davis

Health and Medicine Division Staff

CECILIA MUNDACA SHAH, Director, Forum on Microbial Threats, Board on Global Health
V. AYANO OGAWA, Program Officer, Board on Global Health
T. ANH TRAN, Senior Program Assistant, Board on Global Health
JULIE PAVLIN, Director, Board on Global Health

---

[1] The National Academies of Sciences, Engineering, and Medicine's planning committees are solely responsible for organizing the workshop, identifying topics, and choosing speakers. The responsibility for the published Proceedings of a Workshop rests with the workshop rapporteurs and the institution.

FORUM ON MICROBIAL THREATS[1]

DAVID A. RELMAN (*Chair*), Thomas C. and Joan M. Merigan Professor, Departments of Medicine and of Microbiology and Immunology, Stanford University

JAMES M. HUGHES (*Vice Chair*), Professor of Medicine and Public Health, Rollins School of Public Health, Emory University

LONNIE J. KING (*Vice Chair*), Professor and Dean Emeritus, College of Veterinary Medicine, The Ohio State University

KEVIN ANDERSON, Senior Program Manager, Science and Technology Directorate, U.S. Department of Homeland Security

TIMOTHY BURGESS, Director, Infectious Disease Clinical Research Program, Uniformed Services University of Health Sciences

DENNIS CARROLL, Director, Global Health Security and Development Unit, U.S. Agency for International Development

PETER DASZAK, President, EcoHealth Alliance

JEFFREY S. DUCHIN, Health Officer and Chief, Communicable Disease Epidemiology and Immunization Section for Public Health, Seattle and King County, Washington

EMILY ERBELDING, Deputy Director, Division of AIDS, National Institute of Allergy and Infectious Diseases, National Institutes of Health

MARCOS A. ESPINAL, Director, Department of Communicable Diseases and Health Analysis, Pan American Health Organization

JENNIFER GARDY, Canada Research Chair in Public Health Genomics; Assistant Professor, University of British Columbia

JESSE L. GOODMAN, Professor of Medicine and Infectious Diseases; Director, Center on Medical Product Access, Safety, and Stewardship, Georgetown University

EVA HARRIS, Professor, Division of Infectious Disease and Vaccinology; Director, Center for Global Public Health, University of California, Berkeley

CAROLINE S. HARWOOD, Gerald and Lyn Grinstein Professor of Microbiology, University of Washington

ELIZABETH D. HERMSEN, Head, Global Antimicrobial Stewardship, Merck & Co., Inc.

KENT E. KESTER, Vice President and Head, Translational Science and Biomarkers, Sanofi Pasteur

---

[1] The National Academies of Sciences, Engineering, and Medicine's forums and roundtables do not issue, review, or approve individual documents. The responsibility for the published Proceedings of a Workshop rests with the workshop rapporteurs and the institution.

RIMA F. KHABBAZ, Deputy Director for Infectious Diseases; Director of Office of Infectious Diseases, U.S. Centers for Disease Control and Prevention

MARLO LIBEL, Senior Advisor, Skoll Global Threats Fund

CARMEN T. MAHER, Assistant Surgeon General and Acting Assistant Commissioner for Counterterrorism and Emerging Threats, U.S. Food and Drug Administration

JONNA MAZET, Professor of Epidemiology and Disease Ecology; Executive Director, One Health Institute, School of Veterinary Medicine, University of California, Davis

SALLY A. MILLER, Professor of Plant Pathology and State Extension Specialist for Vegetable Pathology, Ohio Agricultural Research and Development Center, The Ohio State University

SUERIE MOON, Director of Research, Global Health Centre, Graduate Institute of International and Development Studies, Geneva

DAVID NABARRO, Advisor, Health and Sustainability, 4SD–Skills, Systems, and Synergies for Sustainable Development

GEORGE POSTE, Chief Scientist, Complex Adaptive Systems Initiative, Arizona State University, SkySong

KUMANAN RASANATHAN, Coordinator, Health Systems, Office of the World Health Organization Representative in Cambodia, World Health Organization

GARY A. ROSELLE, Chief of Medical Service, Veterans Affairs Medical Center; Director, National Infectious Disease Services, Veterans Health Administration

PETER A. SANDS, Executive Director, The Global Fund to Fight AIDS, Tuberculosis and Malaria

THOMAS W. SCOTT, Distinguished Professor, Department of Entomology and Nematology, University of California, Davis

JAY P. SIEGEL, Retired Chief Biotechnology Officer, Head of Scientific Strategy and Policy, Johnson & Johnson

JAMI TAYLOR, Senior Director, Global Public Health Systems Policy and Partnerships, Johnson & Johnson

PAIGE E. WATERMAN, Lieutenant Colonel, U.S. Army; Director, Translational Medicine Branch, Walter Reed Army Institute of Research

MARY E. WILSON, Clinical Professor of Epidemiology and Biostatistics, School of Medicine, University of California, San Francisco

EDWARD H. YOU, Supervisory Special Agent, Weapons of Mass Destruction Directorate, Federal Bureau of Investigation

National Academies of Sciences, Engineering, and Medicine Staff

CECILIA MUNDACA SHAH, Director, Forum on Microbial Threats, Board on Global Health
V. AYANO OGAWA, Program Officer, Board on Global Health
T. ANH TRAN, Senior Program Assistant, Board on Global Health
JULIE PAVLIN, Director, Board on Global Health

Reviewers

This Proceedings of a Workshop was reviewed in draft form by individuals chosen for their diverse perspectives and technical expertise. The purpose of this independent review is to provide candid and critical comments that will assist the National Academies of Sciences, Engineering, and Medicine in making each published proceedings as sound as possible and to ensure that it meets the institutional standards for quality, objectivity, evidence, and responsiveness to the charge. The review comments and draft manuscript remain confidential to protect the integrity of the process.

We thank the following individuals for their review of this proceedings:

JONNA A. K. MAZET, University of California, Davis
ERIC MINTZ, U.S. Centers for Disease Control and Prevention
THOMAS W. SCOTT, University of California, Davis
ALICE SVERDLIK, International Institute for Environment and Development, London

Although the reviewers listed above provided many constructive comments and suggestions, they were not asked to endorse the content of the proceedings nor did they see the final draft before its release. The review of this proceedings was overseen by **DAVID R. CHALLONER,** University of Florida. He was responsible for making certain that an independent examination of this proceedings was carried out in accordance with standards of the National Academies and that all review comments were carefully considered. Responsibility for the final content rests entirely with the rapporteurs and the National Academies.

Acknowledgments

The Forum on Microbial Threats staff and planning committee deeply appreciate the many valuable contributions from individuals who assisted with this project. The workshop and these proceedings would not be possible without the presenters and discussants at the workshop, who gave so generously of their time and expertise. A full list of the speakers and moderators and their biographical information may be found in Appendix D.

Contents

ACRONYMS AND ABBREVIATIONS   xix

1 INTRODUCTION   1
Workshop Objectives, 2
Organization of the Proceedings of a Workshop, 3

2 PERSPECTIVES ON THE PREVENTION AND CONTROL OF INFECTIOUS DISEASES IN AN URBAN AND INTERCONNECTED WORLD   5
Potential Challenges and Opportunities at the Global Level, 5
Potential Challenges and Opportunities at the Local Level, 12

3 UNDERSTANDING INFECTIOUS DISEASE TRANSMISSION IN URBAN BUILT ENVIRONMENTS   17
The Influence of Slums on Population Health and Microbial Communities, 17
Human Exposure to Microbes in Urban Buildings, 22
Pathways of Pathogen Transmission in Urban Centers, 26
Discussion, 29

4 TRANSLATING CONCEPTUAL MODELS OF INFECTIOUS DISEASE TRANSMISSION AND CONTROL INTO PRACTICE   35
Effect of the West Africa Ebola Virus Disease Outbreak on Other Infectious Diseases, 35

Waterborne Diseases in Dhaka, Bangladesh, 41
Emerging Vector-Borne and Zoonotic Diseases in Brazilian Slums, 45
Tuberculosis Transmission in Cape Town, South Africa, 51
Discussion, 56

5 ACHIEVING SUSTAINABLE AND HEALTH-PROMOTING URBAN BUILT ENVIRONMENTS 61
Global Efforts to Leverage the Sustainable Development Goals to Promote Health, 62
Building an Investment Case for Health-Promoting Urban Environments, 67
Fit-for-Context Water, Sanitation, and Hygiene Interventions, 70
Engaging Communities: From Surveillance to Policy, 76
Discussion, 82

6 BRIDGING DRIVERS AND INTERVENTIONS TO SCALE UP SUCCESSFUL PRACTICES 89
Promoting Health and Health Equity in Low-Income Urban Settings, 90
Scaling Up Successful Practices: Learning from Local Communities, 93
Building the Business Case for Investing in Health-Promoting Urban Environments, 95
Synthesis and General Discussion, 97
Closing Remarks, 103

APPENDIXES
A REFERENCES   105
B WORKSHOP STATEMENT OF TASK   113
C WORKSHOP AGENDA   115
D BIOGRAPHICAL SKETCHES OF WORKSHOP SPEAKERS AND MODERATORS 119

Box and Figures

BOX

5-1 Examples of Methods to Mitigate Infectious Diseases in Slum Environments in India, 68

FIGURES

2-1 Health in relation to other Sustainable Development Goal (SDG) activities and sectors, 7
2-2 Infant and child mortality in rural versus urban areas, 11

3-1 Proportion of group A *Streptococcus* isolate genotypes found at one private clinic (Jorge Valente) and two public clinics (Emergência São Marcos and Quinto Centro) in Salvador, Brazil, 21
3-2 Comparison of exposure in short-range airborne route and large droplet route, showing highest concentrations of inhaled airborne and large droplet exposures within 1.5 meters, 25
3-3 Travel networks of humans and parasites between settlements and regions in Kenya, 28

4-1 Number of probable and confirmed Ebola virus disease (EVD) infections among health care workers in Guinea, Liberia, and Sierra Leone (January 2014 to March 2015), 37

4-2 Co-occurrence of different household-level exposures of high-risk factors for cholera in spatially matched households (matched-sets), 44
4-3 Different barriers facilitate or constrain the flow of pathogens from one species to another, 46
4-4 Modified Wells-Riley equation for estimating annual risk of tuberculosis (TB) infections using number of inhaled TB infectious quanta per year, 52
4-5 Correlation between the mean indoor carbon dioxide concentrations in 62 naturally ventilated classrooms and airflow per person, 55

5-1 Response framework in the World Health Organization's (WHO's) Global Vector Control Response 2017–2030 to reduce the burden and threat of vector-borne diseases affecting humans, 64
5-2 The proportion of urban populations living in slums in African countries, 72
5-3 Global map of the predicted distribution of the *Aedes aegypti* mosquito, 77
5-4 Primary outcomes of cluster randomized controlled trial Camino Verde, a community involvement intervention across two sites in Nicaragua and Mexico, 81

Acronyms and Abbreviations

CDC	U.S. Centers for Disease Control and Prevention
DALY	disability-adjusted life year
ETU	Ebola treatment unit
EVD	Ebola virus disease
MDG	Millennium Development Goal
MTB	*Mycobacterium tuberculosis*
SARS	severe acute respiratory syndrome
SDG	Sustainable Development Goal
SEPA	socializing evidence for participatory action
ORS	oral rehydration solution
PCR	polymerase chain reaction
TB	tuberculosis
UN	United Nations
UN-Habitat	United Nations Human Settlements Programme
WASH	water, sanitation, and hygiene
WHO	World Health Organization

1

Introduction

As the world becomes increasingly urbanized and interconnected, infectious diseases—both existing and emerging—pose a serious and rapidly escalating threat to urban populations if left unaddressed. According to United Nations estimates, the global urban population will top 6 billion by the year 2050, with most of that growth occurring in developing countries (Alirol et al., 2011). Along with this exponential urban growth there has been a concomitant surge in the number of people living in urban and periurban slums, as population pressures cause urban centers to grow upwards and outwards. Today, an estimated one in eight people around the world live in slums, and although the proportion of people living in slums has decreased worldwide over the past 15 years, the absolute number is currently approaching 1 billion people, with no sign of that growth abating (UN-Habitat, 2016a).

The urban built environment includes all physical parts of where humans live and work in a city, such as homes, buildings, streets, open spaces, and infrastructure. The urban built environment is a prime setting for microbial transmission, because just as cities serve as hubs for migration and international travel, components of the urban built environment serve as hubs that drive the transmission of infectious disease pathogens (Alirol et al., 2011). The risk of infectious diseases for many people living in slums is further compounded by their poverty and their surrounding physical and social environment, which is often overcrowded, is prone to physical hazards, and lacks adequate or secure housing and basic infrastructure, including water, sanitation, or hygiene services (Ezeh et al., 2017). These conditions harbor an ideal setting for mosquito vector development and resting sites and the transmission of waterborne diseases. If people in slums do become ill, many of them lack access to health services for treatment. Though slum conditions vary economically and socially across regions and within countries, the populations most at risk will face worsening health consequences if the growth in urban and slum populations is not matched with an increased emphasis on research that brings together disciplines, such as urban planning, public health, environmental health, and social and behavioral sciences. Such action would help further elucidate disease transmission in urban areas and the specific challenges associated with studying and implementing interventions in slums.

WORKSHOP OBJECTIVES

To examine the role of the urban built environment in the emergence and reemergence of infectious diseases that affect human health, the Forum on Microbial Threats at the National Academies of Sciences, Engineering, and Medicine, in collaboration with the Board on Life Sciences, planned the 1.5-day public workshop Urbanization and Slums: New Transmission Pathways of Infectious Diseases in the Built Environment.[1] The following topics were explored during the workshop[2]:

- The formation, function, and interaction of microbial communities in the urban built environment that affect human health;
- Specific urban built environment characteristics, spatial heterogeneity, and land-use patterns, as well as social and behavioral factors (host and vector movement) that may alter vector distribution and increase or facilitate transmission of infectious diseases;
- Critical opportunities, challenges, and knowledge gaps relevant to translating research findings into practical application of shaping urban environments that prevent and mitigate infectious disease outbreaks;
- Innovative strategies, interventions, and policies for creating sustainable and health-promoting urban built environments that consider structural and socioeconomic determinants of diseases;
- Obtaining valid and reliable data to monitor and evaluate implementation and progress of programs and policies; and

---

[1] The planning committee's role was limited to planning the workshop, and the Proceedings of a Workshop was prepared by the workshop rapporteurs as a factual summary of what occurred at the workshop. Statements, recommendations, and opinions expressed are those of individual presenters and participants, and are not necessarily endorsed or verified by the National Academies of Sciences, Engineering, and Medicine, and they should not be construed as reflecting any group consensus.

[2] The full Statement of Task is available in Appendix B.

- Collaboration and coordination mechanisms among various stakeholders and across sectors in urban planning, public policy, public health, animal health, environmental health, microbiology, and social and behavioral sciences.

The 1.5-day workshop was held in Washington, DC, on December 12 and 13, 2017. The workshop was co-chaired by James Hughes, professor of medicine and public health at Emory University Rollins School of Public Health, and Mary Wilson, clinical professor of epidemiology and biostatistics at the University of California, San Francisco. Workshop speakers and discussants contributed perspectives from government, academia, and the private and nonprofit sectors. The workshop featured 2 keynote addresses and 11 speaker presentations over two sessions. During the third session, workshop speakers, forum members, and attendees broke into three groups to discuss set themes related to promotion of health and control of infectious diseases in urban built environments.

ORGANIZATION OF THE PROCEEDINGS OF A WORKSHOP

In accordance with the policies of the National Academies, the workshop did not attempt to establish any conclusions or recommendations about needs and future directions, focusing instead on information presented, questions raised, and improvements recommended by individual workshop participants. Chapter 2 features two keynote presentations that explored potential challenges and opportunities for the prevention and control of infectious diseases in an increasingly urban and interconnected world, from both global and local perspectives. Chapters 3 and 4 include presentations and discussions from session 1 of the workshop, which examined social, physical, environmental, and political drivers of infectious disease transmission in the urban built environment. Specifically, Chapter 3 features presentations that explore the link between slums and adverse health outcomes, routes of pathogen transmission in urban buildings, and pathways of pathogens within, into, and out of urban centers. Chapter 4 features presentations that focus on translating conceptual models into practice, with illustrative examples describing efforts against the Ebola virus disease outbreak in West Africa, waterborne diseases in Bangladesh, Zika and leptospirosis in Brazilian slums, and tuberculosis in Cape Town, South Africa. Chapter 5 covers presentations and discussion from session 2 of the workshop, which examined effective interventions and policies for achieving sustainable and health-promoting urban built environments; presenters described experiences with water, sanitation, and hygiene interventions, with slum upgrading and health promotion in India, and with community engagement against dengue in Mexico and Nicaragua. Chapter 6 explores research gaps to bridge drivers and interventions toward scaling up successful practices, featuring reports from the breakout group moderators and highlights from the large group discussion.

2

Perspectives on the Prevention and Control of Infectious Diseases in an Urban and Interconnected World

During the opening session, two speakers set the stage by exploring current challenges and opportunities for the prevention and control of infectious diseases in an increasingly urban and interconnected world. Christopher Dye, director of strategy, policy, and information at the Office of the Director-General of the World Health Organization (WHO), provided a global perspective on those challenges and opportunities, focusing on how global initiatives like Transforming Our World: The 2030 Agenda for Sustainable Development,[1] commonly known as the Sustainable Development Goals (SDGs), can contribute to countering microbial threats in the urban environment. A local perspective that highlighted the role of slums in global disease transmission was offered by Alex Ezeh, former executive director of the African Population and Health Research Center in Kenya.

POTENTIAL CHALLENGES AND OPPORTUNITIES AT THE GLOBAL LEVEL

The SDGs came into force as a nonbinding international agreement in 2016, consisting of 17 global goals that span 169 specific targets to be

---

[1] The 2030 Agenda for Sustainable Development is available at www.un.org/sustainabledevelopment/development-agenda (accessed January 11, 2018).

achieved by 2030,[2] with the overarching aim of promoting sustainable development by harmonizing the interconnected elements of economic growth, social inclusion, and environmental protection. Christopher Dye, director of strategy, policy, and information at the Office of the Director-General of WHO, explored how the SDGs could contribute to mitigating microbial threats in urban environments, noting the diversity of opinions about the potential impact of the agenda. He suggested that the agenda could indeed serve as a "guiding light" for development, with the proviso that it be treated as an agenda for research—that is, a set of testable ideas—and not as a blueprint for development.

Dye maintained that the SDGs reflect a shift in thinking about health in the context of development. He explained that the antecedent to the SDGs, the Millennium Development Goals (MDGs),[3] were focused on time-limited, vertical programs targeting principal causes of illness and death in low-income countries, with particular focus on communicable diseases and on the major causes of death among women and children. The proposition for development underpinning the SDGs is different, according to Dye, because its focus is on building horizontal, sustainable, and effective health systems to accelerate health gains through treatment and prevention. This includes health systems concerned with public health and the traditional provision of medical and clinical services, he continued, as well as systems that bring health together with agriculture, education, transportation, energy, industry, and other sectors. Dye commended this broader systemic view, but he cautioned that it will require a host of new ideas to succeed in advancing health.

SDG 3 ("good health and well-being") both depends on and contributes to many of the other SDGs, explained Dye. He described how the relationship between health and the urban environment surpasses the binary relationship between SDG 3 and SDG 11 ("sustainable cities and communities"), because the landscape of urban health is also contingent upon goals related to poverty, education, equity, food, energy, industry, and other sectors (see Figure 2-1). This is reflected in another shift in perspective, he said, from a focus on activities organized around the burden of disease and major causes of death worldwide to activities focused on health, but not organized around specific infectious diseases. For example, new activities aimed at setting priorities for improving the urban environment are orga-

---

[2] The 17 SDGs include no poverty; zero hunger; good health and well-being; quality education; gender equality; clean water and sanitation; affordable and clean energy; decent work and economic growth; industry, innovation, and infrastructure; reduced inequalities; sustainable cities and communities; responsible consumption and production; climate action; life below water; life on land; peace, justice, and strong institutions; and partnerships for the goals.

[3] Established in 2000, the MDGs were a set of eight international development goals with targets to be achieved by 2015.

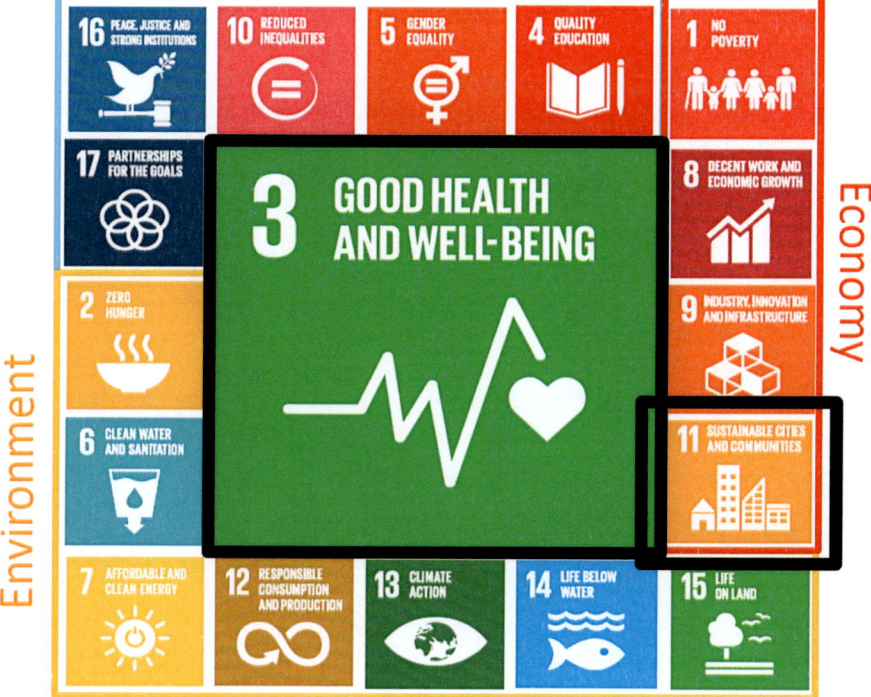

FIGURE 2-1 Health in relation to other Sustainable Development Goal (SDG) activities and sectors.
SOURCES: Dye presentation, December 12, 2017; adapted from WHO, 2017b. Reprinted from *Health in the SDG era,* Copyright (2017).

nized around the processes that underlie developing urban systems, he said, rather than focusing only on specific diseases as causes of illness and death.

Specifically, Dye reported that the United Nations Human Settlements Programme (UN-Habitat) reviewed 5,000 initiatives from 140 countries to identify best practices for developing the urban environment, and set forth priorities, including slum upgrading; water, sanitation, and hygiene services; housing; urban governance; urban planning; and urban economy.

Dye characterized the persistent decline in mortality among children under 5 years of age as a spectacular success of the previous half century. He explained that, although rates declined across high-, middle-, and low-income countries throughout this period, there was an accelerated decline in low-income countries, where the mortality rate began to converge with rates for middle- and high-income countries between 1990 and 2015. Dye noted that this period of convergence was largely coincident with the MDG era, but suggested that much of the success achieved during that era was driven by factors that were not explicitly taken into account at the time. He cited an analysis that found that only around half of the overall reduction in child mortality was attributable to health services and direct medical interventions, such as vaccines, oral rehydration, or antibiotic treatment (Kuruvilla et al., 2014). The remaining proportion was attributed to efforts addressing deeper causes and risks, including reducing population fertility; increasing female political and socioeconomic participation and primary education; improving environmental factors; economic development; and decreasing income equality. According to Dye, the reduction in child mortality is inexplicable without these primary prevention factors, which can be roughly aligned with various SDGs. Dye maintained that forging links between health and the other SDGs would promote the development of health systems that are oriented not only toward treatment but also toward cost-effective prevention.

Bolstering Systems That Promote Health

Dye explored some of the characteristics of systems that serve to promote health and well-being, which he discussed in two categories. With regard to the first category, he explained that sustainable systems for health require active work on health across all sectors of government, and such systems should provide universal health coverage to the population. With respect to the second category, he outlined five properties of effective systems fostered by the SDGs: affordable, equitable, measurable, testable, and sustainable. Dye framed his discussion of bolstering systems to promote health using these two categories.

Sustainable Systems for Health

Dye reported that the profile of health in the development sphere is on the rise, which is a legacy of the MDG era being propelled in the SDG era. Discussions taking place at the highest levels of international organizations are being mirrored at the level of many national governments, he said, and health matters are increasingly considered matters for the whole of government and not just the ministry of health. Developments in intersectoral work on health are also under way, said Dye. He reflected that 30 years ago he had to stop his work on the biology of leishmaniasis transmission in the Amazon,[4] because lack of interest in the disease frustrated his efforts to

---

[4] Leishmaniasis is a parasitic disease transmitted by bites of phlebotomine sand flies that can cause sores on the skin or affect internal organs.

translate his biology research findings into real public health actions. However, he said, this changed substantially when leishmaniasis was classified as a neglected tropical disease, raising its profile and driving the development of new control strategies, such as canine vaccines to prevent transmission of visceral leishmaniasis to humans.

Years ago, he remarked, urbanization was not even considered a factor, despite observations that there was no leishmaniasis in settlements on the edge of towns, where people lived in different types of housing than areas affected by the disease. Today, it is well established that good housing engenders multiple health benefits and is part of the solution for leishmaniasis and other issues, said Dye, because poor-quality housing and neglected peridomestic environments are risks for vector-borne and other illnesses. He attributed this development in part to the broadening of perspective the SDGs are bringing to the fore, which is driving innovation in housing design to strengthen vector control. However, he warned that, despite the well-known broader and sustainable benefits of quality housing for a population, efforts to improve housing are often neglected in favor of other interventions. According to Dye, this is because poor housing is generally seen as a relatively weak risk factor for vector-borne and other illnesses, so it is often sidelined for efforts focusing exclusively on disease-specific interventions (for example, bed nets for malaria control).

Dye suggested channeling research and funding toward better quantitative systems analyses of the interactions among different SDGs and of different potential interventions. He cited a study that analyzed the relationship between SDG 3 and SDG 11, which found a key interaction between housing and respiratory disease (Griggs et al., 2017). This type of work may serve as a starting point for addressing diseases in the urban environment, he noted, but advised that deeper, more detailed work will be needed to identify connections that can be leveraged to devise better disease control programs.

Dye described a study he co-authored on tuberculosis (TB) to illustrate the complexities at play in this type of analysis (Dye et al., 2011). The study began with the observation that undernutrition is a risk factor for TB, yet overnutrition can also be a risk factor for TB via the onset of diabetes mellitus—Dye termed this a "vicious triangle." Both undernutrition and overnutrition are affected by aging, urbanization, and other potential cofactors, he said, so he and his colleagues analyzed the interacting factors to identify the most important drivers of TB in populations in India and Korea. They concluded that demographic factors were the strongest drivers, rather than diabetes or nutrition per se.

Properties of Effective Systems Fostered by the SDGs

Dye explained that universal health coverage is a component of sustainable systems for health as well as a contributor to the properties of effective systems fostered by the SDGs, including affordability and equity. Universal health coverage is a matter of economics as well as equity, he maintained. He reported that as of December 2017, around 12 percent of the population spend more than 10 percent of their household budget on health services, which risks pushing them into poverty (WHO and World Bank, 2017). Although universal health coverage has been called an "affordable dream" by economist Amartya Sen, Dye warned that affording it will be difficult under a number of circumstances. He explained that, per WHO statistics, public expenditure on health as a fraction of gross domestic product has been rising worldwide as well as in low-income countries, albeit slowly. He added that rates of out-of-pocket expenditure as a percentage of health expenditure—which drives people into poverty—have been falling, but also slowly. The question at hand, said Dye, is whether these slow trends will continue or if mechanisms could be implemented to bend these curves upwards or downwards.

Urbanization is the catalyst for various dilemmas of inequity, said Dye. Many of the poorest people migrate to slums because the circumstances there are often better for them than in rural areas, he explained. For example, he reported that, in many countries, rates of infant mortality are higher in rural environments than in urban environments (see Figure 2-2). He noted that, although rates of child mortality tend to be better for poorer people in urban versus rural areas, the inequalities between the poorest and richest people are even greater in urban areas. "Health is better, but inequality is greater too: that is an urban dilemma we need to resolve," said Dye.

Despite media attention to mounting income inequality worldwide, he remarked, WHO statistics suggest that health equality is steadily improving and that the health gap is slowly narrowing between poor and rich people in low- and middle-income countries. He described a WHO analysis on the composite coverage index for a set of health services that used Demographic and Health Survey data from 42 low- and middle-income countries over roughly 10 years (Dye, 2008).[5] It revealed greater relative improvements in the composite coverage index for the poorest quintile versus the richest quintile. He indicated that while inequity in health seems to be declining based on this analysis and others, the real problem is that it is declining too slowly.

---

[5] The health services include family planning; antenatal care; skilled birth attendance; diphtheria, pertussis, and tetanus (three doses) immunization; and care seeking for children with pneumonia.

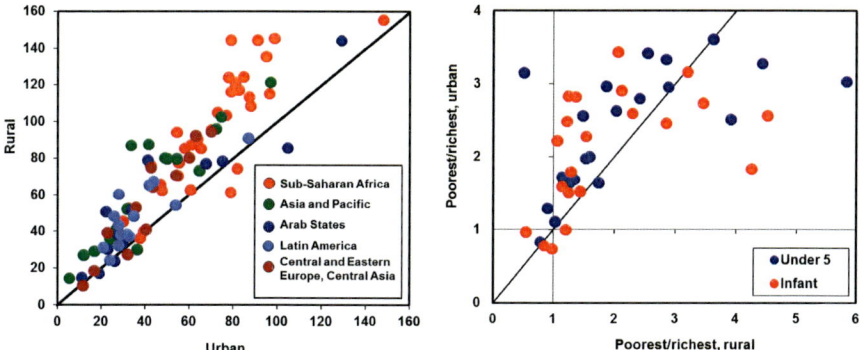

FIGURE 2-2 Infant and child mortality in rural versus urban areas.
Left: Infant mortality under 1 year of age per 1,000 live births tends to be higher in rural than in urban areas.
Right: The ratio of child mortalities (infant and under 5 years of age) in the poorest 20 percent of families to the richest 20 percent tends to be higher in urban than in rural areas.
SOURCES: Dye presentation, December 12, 2017; Dye, 2008. Modified from Dye, C. 2008. Health and urban living. *Science* 319(5864):766-769 with permission.

Although it can be useful to summarize national averages on statistics, said Dye, it is also important to analyze the data in a more detailed, disaggregated way to understand more about who is being left behind—that is, the poorest people in the lowest quintile. Achieving universal health coverage will require more sophisticated measurements and analyses of statistics to understand where the disadvantages lie, he said, and to understand the determinants of socioeconomic circumstances.

To describe the challenge of improving equity, Dye used the case of the 2017 Grenfell Tower fire disaster in central London, England, in which 80 people were killed in a residential tower fire. The tower is in a borough of London where some of the poorest and richest people in the country live alongside each other, he said, and the issue of equity has been the crux of debate and backlash surrounding the circumstances that led to the disaster. Dye explained that this London borough has had essentially the same patterns of rich and poor areas since 1900, highlighting the difficulty in making headway against deeply entrenched social inequities.

Dye concluded by commenting briefly on sustainability and financing of the 2030 agenda. National health accounts are used as the principal measure of how much is spent on health, he noted, but spending is only counted if health is its primary purpose. He cautioned that this is at odds with the SDG agenda's central ethos of integrating various sectors that have attendant health benefits—such as agriculture, education, and transportation—because spending in those sectors is not counted in financing statistics. Dye used funding statistics from the Ebola virus disease (EVD) epidemic of 2014 to discuss sustainability in the context of how funds are invested. Around $9 billion was pledged and $6 billion disbursed overall, he reported, with more than $4.5 billion of those disbursed funds spent on the rapid response to contain the immediate threat. However, he noted that the amount of disbursed funds spent on response dwarfs the amount invested in improving sustainability through recovery efforts (around $1 billion) and through research and development (around $200 million). Dye emphasized that greater investment in sustainability through systems strengthening, research, and development will be critical for preventing and mitigating the threat of future epidemics and pandemics. He said that, in his experience, the value of investing in research is often questioned by those outside the research community; he urged the research community to continue to impress the value of ongoing and increased investment in research on other sectors. Dye reiterated that the SDGs could serve as a transformative guiding light for development work geared toward sustainability, but only if the goals are treated as testable hypotheses and supported by a closely linked research agenda that can measure the benefits of the SDG approach.

POTENTIAL CHALLENGES AND OPPORTUNITIES AT THE LOCAL LEVEL

Alex Ezeh, former executive director of the African Population and Health Research Center in Kenya, opened by remarking that the dynamics of slums are markedly different from those of urban processes as a whole. The growing recognition that slums have unique characteristics that need to be better understood, he continued, is also garnering attention to the role of slums in pathogen transmission and epidemics worldwide. He predicted that as the world becomes increasingly urbanized, effective control of infectious diseases on the global front will hinge upon a better understanding of disease dynamics in urban settings. By 2050, he added, the global population is projected to increase by 2.2 billion people, most of whom will be living in urban areas in low- and middle-income countries.

The challenges faced by people living in slums are tantamount to the challenges of the shared physical and social environments in which they live, remarked Ezeh. The importance of space to people living in slums was underscored by a recent series in *The Lancet* on slum health (Ezeh et al., 2017; Lilford et al., 2017). For people living in slums, he explained, it is not just an individual's household poverty status that matters but also the context within which the individual is living—the neighborhood effects. He added that poverty in and of itself is not a good measure of health in urban areas; given the complex dynamics of urban environments, the drivers of health for people living in slums have less to do with individual wealth compared to the environment in which they live.

Measuring Slums: Statistics Versus Geography

Ezeh pointed out an inconsistency between how slums are measured statistically and what slums actually are. When people think of slums, he said, they typically picture a specific space or geographic location. However, he noted that current estimates and statistics about slums in low- and middle-income countries are derived from UN-Habitat data, which do not characterize slums as specific places. He explained that the following criteria are used to identify people living in slums instead: groups of people or households that lack access to safe water, sanitation, and other infrastructure; people who have insecure tenure within the urban space; and people living in high-density settings (defined as three or more people in the same sleeping room) (UN-Habitat, 2006). Ezeh observed that because estimates based on these data do not refer to the specific geographic locations commonly considered to be slums in low- and middle-income countries, the practical value of these estimates is not entirely clear.

Rising slum populations driven by urbanization in low- and middle-income countries are a major challenge for development going forward, according to Ezeh. Although there has been a significant drop in the proportion of people who live in slums globally since 1990, he said, the absolute number has grown by about 200 million people to roughly 1 billion living in slums today (UN-Habitat, 2016a). In sub-Saharan Africa, the proportion has declined from 70 percent to 56 percent, he added, but the number of people living in slums has more than doubled from about 93 million to about 200 million (UN-Habitat, 2016a). Progress is being made toward helping countries develop better practices for identifying people who live in slums and begin creating strategies for how to help address the specific issues and challenges faced by those populations, said Ezeh. For example, a 2017 meeting in Bellagio, Italy, on slum identification convened representatives from international agencies and the national governments of low- and middle-income countries to strategize about how to deal with slums as a specific development challenge (UN-Habitat, 2017). One objective of the meeting, he noted, was to work toward recognizing slums as geographic entities—with people living in them—in order to capture more accurate information in national data systems and global report estimates.

Understanding the Importance of Slum Health

Ezeh emphasized that better understanding slum health is important, because rural areas and urban areas have fundamentally different health risks, solutions, and opportunities to intervene within their respective settings. He added that there are also distinct dynamics at play in slums versus nonslum areas within urban settings. To highlight the relevance of slum health in global disease transmission and in understanding global health in the 21st century, he outlined five issues:

1. Health risks,
2. Health determinants,
3. Health outcomes,
4. Global interconnectedness, and
5. Urban inequities.

Ezeh explained that many of the health risks faced by slum residents are driven by their environments, such as overcrowding, poor garbage disposal, poor toilet facilities, lack of affordable clean water, and poor drainage. These are constant features within slums in many low- and middle-income countries, he noted. Furthermore, slum residents are inequitably and systematically excluded from health amenities and services in urban areas that are readily available to nonslum residents, he explained. This is not usually the case in rural areas, he said, where most people have access to the same basic health services regardless of their wealth status.

Slum residents and the urban poor face health risks that are driven by environmental determinants, Ezeh maintained, and these determinants of health may be very different from those in other settings. To illustrate how the challenges and constraints of life in slums can be obfuscated by statistical averages for entire urban areas, he presented data from a longitudinal health and demographic surveillance system carried out in the slums of Nairobi from 2003 to 2016 (Beguy et al., 2015). The leading cause of death in adults 15 years of age and older was TB for both men and women, he reported, but injuries were the second most common cause of death for men (31 percent), which he attributed to the slum setting. For children under 5 years of age, the leading cause of death was acute respiratory infection (38.6 percent of males and 32.5 percent of females), he reported. Ezeh also attributed this to the environment, noting that children under 5 years of age spend much of their time inside homes where indoor air pollution is rampant.

Ezeh explained that not only can health risks and determinants of health differ depending on rural, urban, and slum settings, but health outcomes can also differ considerably depending on the environmental context. These differences need to be analyzed more precisely in order to intervene effectively, he argued, citing data comparing mortality rates for infants and children under 5 years of age in different settings in Kenya (APHRC, 2002; Government of Kenya, 2004). Children under 5 years of age in slum households have a 30 percent higher mortality rate than children in rural areas, according to a representative survey of slum households in Nairobi. He added that the difference in mortality rates in slums versus nonslum urban areas is much larger than the difference in the mortality rates between urban and rural areas. However, he cautioned that these estimates and indicators of health outcomes in urban areas may be based on data that do not accurately capture slum communities or represent how their health outcomes are distinct from the broader urban setting. He explained that in the city of Nairobi, for example, an estimated 55 percent of the population actually lives in slums, but national survey data indicate that only 20 percent of the people live in slums.

The urbanization of infectious disease epidemics underscores the role of global interconnectedness as a driver of health worldwide, said Ezeh. Similarly, he noted that outbreaks of EVD were confined to small, remote areas in different African countries prior to the 2014 epidemic, but the epidemic precipitated when it reached three capital cities in West Africa. Interconnectedness exacerbates disease transmission risks outside of households, Ezeh said. He reported that contact-tracing data from the 2009 H1N1 influenza epidemic in China revealed that 44 percent of traced close contacts of index cases were passengers on the same flight, 23 percent were at school or work, and 6 percent were service people in public places (Pang et al., 2011).

Low- and middle-income countries have massive urban inequities that also play a role in driving the transmission of infectious disease, said Ezeh. He explained that disease transmission can be accelerated by the lack of physical and social distance between socioeconomic groups in low- and middle-income countries, where there tend to be huge numbers of people who span diverse socioeconomic milieus every day in their work and homes (for example, domestic staff, hospitality workers, gardeners, cleaners, security staff). He described how the 2017 cholera outbreak in Nairobi became an emergency when it stretched beyond the slums and into the five-star hotels and restaurants, transmitted by workers who became infected in the slums where they live. Ezeh contrasted this proximity between socioeconomic groups with a situation in high-income countries, where welfare systems in place may create physical and social distance between socioeconomic groups because the poorest people may be systematically excluded from the workplace.

Ezeh predicted that slums will emerge as the major nexus between the urban and rural, between the formal and informal, and between the local and global. Given that the slums of low- and middle-income countries are the birthplace of many global epidemics, he maintained, slum health cannot continue to be ignored if efforts to control disease and infection on the global front are to succeed.

3

Understanding Infectious Disease Transmission in Urban Built Environments

Session 1 of the workshop focused on potential social, physical, environmental, and political drivers of infectious disease transmission in the urban built environment. During the first half of the session, moderated by Maria Gloria Dominguez-Bello of New York University School of Medicine, presenters explored how infectious diseases are transmitted in urban built environments. Lee Riley, professor and head of the Infectious Diseases and Vaccinology Division at the University of California, Berkeley, discussed how characteristics of slums can contribute to adverse health outcomes. Yuguo Li, professor of mechanical engineering at the University of Hong Kong, described some of the mechanisms and implications of human exposure to microbes in urban buildings, with a focus on the three major routes of respiratory infection transmission. David Smith, professor of global health at the University of Washington, explored the migration and movement of pathogens through pathways within, into, and out of urban centers, highlighting a project that mapped the transmission of malaria using cellular phone data in Kenya.

THE INFLUENCE OF SLUMS ON POPULATION HEALTH AND MICROBIAL COMMUNITIES

Framing the issues surrounding slum health, Lee Riley, professor and head of the Infectious Diseases and Vaccinology Division at the University of California, Berkeley, noted that the topic has been on the table for more than a decade, ever since the United Nations Human Settlements Programme (UN-Habitat) released a report in 2003 describing the conditions of slums worldwide (UN-Habitat, 2003). The report was the first formal documentation of issues related to urban slums, he said, and it helped to establish an official definition of urban slums, with demographic, spatial, economic, legal, and social indicators for the 1 billion slum residents worldwide at the time. He explained that the report addressed life expectancy and mortality in children under 5 years of age, access to improved water sources and sanitation, and slum upgrading and poverty reduction programs. However, the report did not address health indicators, Riley said, perhaps because measures of health burden can be difficult to assess.

Riley remarked that the term *slum* historically has a negative connotation, although it continues to be accepted terminology by international organizations such as the United Nations (UN). According to the UN operational definition of a slum,[1] a slum is a human settlement with inadequate access to safe water, inadequate access to sanitation and other infrastructure, poor structural quality of housing, overcrowding, and insecure residential status. By that operational definition, the number of people living in slums has progressively increased over the years, Riley reported. According to a 2016 UN-Habitat report, the proportion of urban residents living in slums in developing countries has decreased, but the absolute number of people has steadily increased (UN-Habitat, 2016a).

Riley explained that in Chennai, India, and in many large cities around the world, the extremely rich and poor live in adjacent neighborhoods, with slums and luxury high-rise residential buildings standing in stark contrast to one another. Despite their proximity, he said, slum residents require a different type of health care from residents of wealthier areas. To illustrate this, he described the Paraisópolis neighborhood in São Paulo, Brazil, where a fence separates the slums from the affluent residential areas. He said that residents of both areas are affected by infectious diseases, including tuberculosis (TB), HIV/AIDS, sexually transmitted infections, influenza, sepsis, urinary tract infections, hospital infections, and pharyngitis. However, he said that residents of the slum area are additionally susceptible to diseases that rarely affect residents of the adjacent affluent area, such as leptospirosis, meningitis, hepatitis (A, B, and C), vaccine-preventable diseases, multidrug-resistant TB, rheumatic heart disease, advanced stage cervical carcinoma, and microcephaly. Quoting architect and urban planner Gita Verma, who said that "the root cause of urban slums is not in urban poverty but in urban wealth," Riley emphasized that it is urban wealth—rather than poverty—that is determining health outcomes in the slums (Verma, 2002).`

---

[1] The definition was created by a UN Expert Group in Nairobi in 2000.

Potential Contribution of Slums to Adverse Health Outcomes

To explore the science around the issue of slum health and in terms of infectious diseases, Riley examined slum-specific factors that contribute to adverse health outcomes. He framed the discussion using three components of the UN's definition of slums: inadequate access to sanitation and other infrastructure, insecure residential status, and overcrowding.

Riley explained that, in slums, inadequate access to sanitation and other infrastructure drives multiple adverse health outcomes. Increased rat density contributes to transmission of leptospirosis and typhus, he said, and open sewers contribute to hookworm, leptospirosis, diarrhea, cholera, dengue, malaria, hepatitis, and growth retardation. He said that suboptimal schools are associated with poor health education and poor nutrition; he added that undernutrition and obesity are associated with infectious disease outcomes. He reported that inappropriate and inadequate health services both contribute to poor vaccine coverage, maternal health complications, underutilization of health services, rheumatic heart disease, suicide, drug-resistant TB, and chronic diseases, such as hypertension and diabetes. Lack of residential infrastructure, such as street lighting and public bathrooms, is linked to violence against women and intentional injuries, he added. Injuries are the biggest contributor to poor health outcomes in young adult males, he said, and if people do not die immediately of intentional injuries, they often die of infectious complications of those injuries.

Riley described how insecure residential status and overcrowding are also associated with adverse health outcomes among many slum dwellers. He explained that people with insecure residential status—people living in informal tenure without a title deed—often lack representation, which could contribute to their exclusion from health care services and from having a voice in vital decisions that affect community health outcomes. He added that people who are evicted often lack access to health care services, schooling, and employment. Many people born in slum communities are not officially registered, he said, which excludes them from health care and education services as well. Furthermore, people living in such conditions are often exposed to toxic chemicals, he said, which can lead to poisoning, respiratory diseases, and cancer. He noted that the major causes of death in developing countries are infectious diseases. Finally, he suggested that low health service utilization compounds the problem by contributing to chronic diseases; unwanted pregnancy; sexually transmitted infections, including HIV; and illnesses related to substance abuse. Riley said that overcrowding in slums also engenders a host of opportunities for transmission of diseases, including TB, respiratory diseases, pharyngitis, meningitis, scabies, superinfections of the skin, acute glomerulonephritis, rheumatic heart disease, and Zika virus infection and its congenital consequences. Riley focused more closely on two diseases—rheumatic heart disease and Zika virus disease—to describe how slum conditions can drive transmission.

Rheumatic Heart Disease

Rheumatic heart disease is an immunologically mediated chronic complication of group A streptococcal pharyngitis. Past World Health Organization (WHO) estimates suggested that prevalence of the disease peaks in young adults between the ages of 24 and 35 years (WHO, 2005). However, Riley reported that studies from Brazil have suggested that the mean age of severe complications of the disease has decreased. According to a study in Salvador, the median age at which children developed congestive heart failure and stroke was 12 years (Câmara et al., 2002), and a later study reported a median age as low as 9 years (Câmara et al., 2004).

To illustrate how the diversity of microbial communities for the same disease, in the same city, can affect health interventions and outcomes, Riley described a study examining the genetic distribution of group A *Streptococcus* carried out in three clinics in the city of Salvador, Brazil (Tartof et al., 2010). Two of the clinics included in the study were public and predominantly served children living in urban slums (São Marcos and Quinto Centro), while the other was a private clinic (Jorge Valente). The investigators examined the genetic distribution of group A *Streptococcus* in children with sore throat and generated Simpson's Diversity Index scores capturing the variation of the number of *emm* gene sequences at each clinic. Riley reported that the diversity index for the isolates from the children who attended the private clinic was 0.92, which is almost identical to the diversity index for high-income countries according to a systematic review of global *emm* type distribution (Steer et al., 2009). The diversity indices for genotypes from children treated in the two slum clinics (Quinto Centro: 0.97; São Marcos: 0.96) were similar to those found in African countries (0.981) and Pacific region countries (0.979) (Steer et al., 2009; Tartof et al., 2010).

Riley explained that the investigators also examined the proportion of group A *Streptococcus* isolate genotypes found at each of the clinics (Tartof et al., 2010) (see Figure 3-1). The two most common isolates at the private clinic (Jorge Valente) were *emm*12.0 and *emm*1.0, representing 36 percent of isolates; he noted these are also the two most common isolates found in high-income countries (Steer et al., 2009). He said that in the two slum clinics, *emm*12.0 and *emm*1.0 represented lower proportions (São Marcos: 21 percent; Quinto Centro: 14 percent) (Tartof et al., 2010). In comparison, those two isolates account for less than 10 percent in African regions (Steer et al., 2009). Riley highlighted these findings because *emm*12.0 and *emm*1.0 are included in the 26-valent experimental vaccine for group A

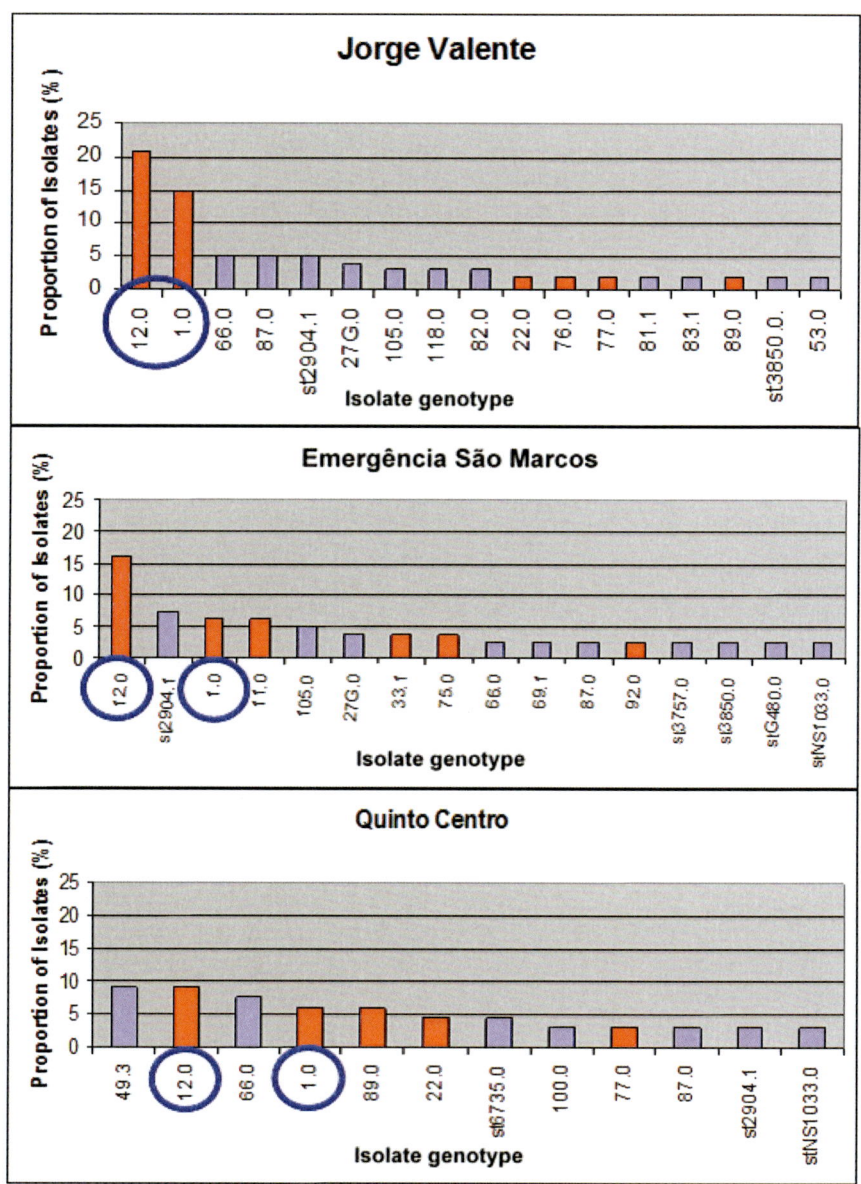

FIGURE 3-1 Proportion of group A *Streptococcus* isolate genotypes found at one private clinic (Jorge Valente) and two public clinics (Emergência São Marcos and Quinto Centro) in Salvador, Brazil.
NOTE: Orange bars are isolates that are included in the 26-valent experimental vaccine for group A *Streptococcus*; purple bars are isolates that are not included.
SOURCES: Riley presentation, December 12, 2017; data from Tartof et al., 2010.

Streptococcus. If the vaccine were administered in Salvador, said Riley, then it would be more efficacious among children in private clinics than children who attend clinics in slums. There is much discussion of disparities in living conditions, he added, but disparities exist down to the cellular level. He maintained that developing better vaccines will require better understanding of the biology of the disease.

Zika Virus Disease

Riley touched on Zika virus infection and its congenital consequences to illustrate another case of how slum conditions, such as overcrowding, inadequate safe water supply, and poor quality housing, can drive high levels of virus transmission. Mosquitoes that thrive in communities living in overcrowded conditions increase the risk of human infection, he explained, so people living in slums are more likely to be exposed to diverse virus populations than people who live in more affluent, less overcrowded areas. It is hypothesized that this may be one mechanism for the higher occurrence of the microcephaly in the congenital Zika syndrome seen among people living in slums, he added. In February 2016, WHO declared a public health emergency of international concern because of the congenital syndrome in newborns of pregnant women infected by Zika, he said, but declared an end to that status later in the same year. Brazil also declared an end to the public health emergency of the Zika epidemic in early 2017, said Riley, but he emphasized that the families of children affected by microcephaly have only just begun to deal with the consequences.

Riley concluded by arguing that we must take immediate steps to formally recognize the existence of this population and not rely solely on achieving the UN Sustainable Development Goals (SDGs). He suggested that people in positions of influence in national governments should prioritize these efforts. He called for working with the residents of slums to assess burdens of disease in slum populations and for identifying and implementing novel interventions specifically designed for slums. To develop new metrics, he suggested that precision public health research should measure the biological, sociological, and environmental determinants of disease.

HUMAN EXPOSURE TO MICROBES IN URBAN BUILDINGS

Yuguo Li, professor of mechanical engineering at the University of Hong Kong, provided an overview of the mechanisms and implications of human exposure to microbes in urban buildings. He began by introducing the three major routes of respiratory infection transmission: through the air people breathe (airborne route), through the surfaces they touch (fomite route), and through other people they meet (close-contact route). He noted that this concept is centuries old.[2] In an urban setting, he explained, there are a huge number of opportunities for transmission as people go about their day in their homes, on public transport, and in offices, classrooms, restaurants, shops, and theaters. He added that transmission can take place through the air in the indoor air network or through close contact with other people by touching them or talking to them, or through fomites (Gao et al., 2016). Fomites are shared surfaces that can harbor and transmit infection. Transmission can take place through short-range or long-range routes, said Li. He explained that short routes involve close contact of less than 1.5 meters with large droplets (> 100 micrometers) transmitted through the air or via direct touching. He said that long-range routes—more than 1.5 meters—involve small droplets, droplet nuclei, or aerosols (< 5 micrometers) transmitted through the air or through contact with fomites (Wei and Li, 2016).

Airborne Route of Transmission

Li explained that the airborne route of transmission involves exposure to fine droplet nuclei exhaled by another person; these droplet nuclei can travel long distances. During the severe acute respiratory syndrome (SARS) nosocomial outbreak in Hong Kong in 2003, Li and his colleagues suggested that the virus transmission was airborne, at least for that particular outbreak (Li et al., 2005). He said that it is difficult to understand why in other outbreaks the virus transmission does not appear to be airborne. Once aerosols become airborne, he added, they are affected by ventilation and airflows in indoor spaces. However, he noted that technologies exist for modern buildings to help engineers improve ventilation and airflows to mitigate transmission (Zhang and Li, 2012). While strategies are available for modern buildings, he noted, there have been few studies about the air quality in slums. He added that ventilation rate is a basic parameter that is not measured or governed by the types of laws and regulations that govern water quality, for example.

Fomite Route of Transmission

The fomite route of transmission involves exposure from touching contaminated inanimate surfaces (fomites), said Li. To illustrate how quickly a virus can be transmitted through the fomite route, he described a study

---

[2] Girolamo Fracastoro (1478–1553) posited that "contagion is an infection that passes from one thing to another" and suggested three routes of transmission: by direct contact, through inanimate objects, and via air.

that investigated an outbreak of norovirus on an airplane in 2009. Of 118 passengers on the plane, 22 became infected, the majority of whom were seated on the aisles (Kirking et al., 2010). Li outlined three possibilities as to why the aisle seat passengers had a greater infection risk through the fomite route: people touch the aisle seats more often than others; crew members have more access to those seats; and/or passengers seated in the aisle may tend to use the toilets more often, where contaminated microbes are prevalent.

Researchers are still working to understand how surfaces become contaminated, said Li. He explained that the simplest version of the fomite route is transmission of a virus from one surface to another through touching. He described a potential model for contact particle transfer that has been developed by one of his colleagues: the trap and pull-off mechanism. First, the particle is trapped by the real touch area through friction (electric contact), he said, and then the particle can be transferred to another surface, depending on which surface has the highest adhesion force. He suggested that this sort of model might potentially help engineers to develop better surfaces for avoiding particle transfer.

Li said that transmission through the fomite route is fast—as fast as the airborne route—because the so-called surface touch network grows logistically and governs this rapid transmission. He explained that after a half-day on an airplane, for example, all of the touch surfaces are connected: the first one is touched by a few people, each person can touch multiple surfaces, and each surface is touched by multiple people. Within three to five generations, all the surfaces are touched. He added that if a person moves to another space while carrying a contaminant, a new surface touch network is formulated (Lei et al., 2017).

Close-Contact Route of Transmission

Exposure through the close-contact route occurs in proximity to the index patient, explained Li. He added that this route has at least three short-range subroutes: large droplets, airborne, and surface touching, such as hand shaking, body touch, or fomite (Liu et al., 2017; Xie et al., 2007) (see Figure 3-2). He added that a virus can move from one place to another through close-contact airborne transmission, which cannot be avoided. A surgical mask can help prevent transmission of large droplets in close contact, he said, but neither general ventilation nor surgical masks can prevent close-contact airborne transmission (less than 1.5 meters). He suggested that new technology is needed to better control short-range airborne transmission.

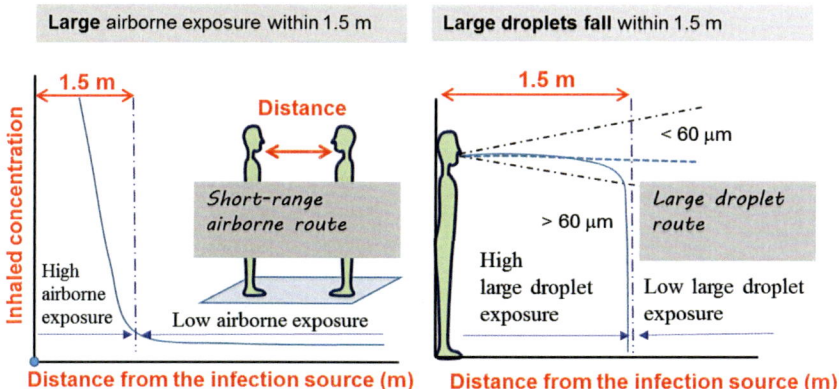

FIGURE 3-2 Comparison of exposure in short-range airborne route and large droplet route, showing highest concentrations of inhaled airborne and large droplet exposures within 1.5 meters.
NOTE: m = meter; μm = micrometer.
SOURCE: Li presentation, December 12, 2017.

Potential Challenges and Knowledge Gaps

Li outlined a set of potential challenges and knowledge gaps with respect to the mechanisms and implications of human exposure to microbes in indoor buildings. For instance, "separating" a particular transmission route from a multiroute process is central to animal tests, outbreak analyses, and other purposes, but it is difficult to separate the three transmission routes (Dick et al., 1987). He added that, although it is relatively easy to separate the airborne routes, it is relatively challenging to separate close-contact routes because of the difficulty of determining the source of inhaled air. He noted that the fomite route may be easier to separate, but there is not a way to do it yet. He reported that there are no field data on indoor air networks and surface touch networks, although some data on close-contact networks have been captured. Another challenge, according to Li, is the rapid evolution of social contact that is being driven by mass travel and rapid urbanization in the built environment. Despite many studies on the microbiome, he said, there is a lack of data about how microbes actually get into mass transit environments, office environments, and homes. He suggested that better understanding of the three routes of transmission will be helpful in addressing this need for data.

Li outlined three knowledge gaps from his perspective: understanding human behavior in buildings, understanding the contribution of individual transmission routes, and the lack of mechanistic models. Addressing the first gap, said Li, will require gathering more detailed data on microscale human behavior to construct models of how humans interact with each other and how they interact with surfaces in a room or building. To better understand surface touch behavior, he suggested creating detailed spatial and temporal profiles that capture data about who touches what surface, for how long (in seconds), in what sequence, with what amount of touch pressure, in what contact area, and so forth. However, he noted that there are ethical concerns to obtaining such behavioral data. He suggested that better understanding the microscale will require new technology, such as rapid indoor positioning systems, body part recognition, and surface recognition systems.

The second gap highlighted by Li is the lack of data and knowledge on the individual route contribution to infection. He suggested identifying effective study designs to carry out individual route studies or human challenge investigations and noted that a number of ferret studies on airborne transmission in the recent literature were unable to demonstrate that large droplet and airborne transmission are separated (Belser et al., 2016; Herfst et al., 2012). He explained that ferret cage studies make it almost impossible to separate out close contact and questioned whether it would be possible to design a better human challenge study. The third gap Li identified was the lack of mechanistic-based pandemic models that could be used to predict the effect of different interventions, to inform policy, and to analyze outbreaks. He attributed this gap to the lack of data on parameters, such as surface survival, fomite-hand transfer rates, dose-response parameters, nose/eye touching frequency, and building data, such as window/door openings.

PATHWAYS OF PATHOGEN TRANSMISSION IN URBAN CENTERS

David Smith, professor of global health at the University of Washington, explored several pathways through which pathogens can be transmitted within, into, and out of urban centers. He noted humans in particular generally carry cell phones with them when they move around, enabling measurement of how often and how far people move. He explained that every time a person makes or receives a call or adds money to their phone, or when their phone pings a cell tower, that transaction is logged, creating a record of where people are at various points in time. He described how cell phone data have been used to investigate pathways of pathogen transmission in Kenya, in combination with other data from the Malaria Atlas Project,[3] which maps how malaria parasites are distributed in the country.

---

[3] The Malaria Atlas Project is available at map.ox.ac.uk (accessed March 14, 2018).

Mapping Malaria Transmission in Kenya

Smith's presentation focused on a study aimed at understanding the human mobility component of malaria transmission in Kenya (Wesolowski et al., 2012). He described how the investigators were able to collect call data records from 15 million anonymized cell phone users in Kenya over approximately 1 year. He explained that around 12,000 cell towers are scattered across Kenya, with most of the users being served by a single cell phone company that facilitated the data collection. He described how the investigators mapped the country's urban areas, densely inhabited buffer settlements surrounding urban areas, and cell tower locations, and then assigned each region a relative risk for malaria. The mode of each unique user's identifier was considered that user's home location, he said, which was used to determine how often users moved away from home and where they moved.

The investigators also tried to map a network of people's contacts at the country level, Smith said. He explained that, to simplify the task of dealing with such a massive and complex data set, the investigators tried to identify communities. Within a network concept, he said, people who belong to the same community tend to be more closely connected to other people in that community than they are to anyone outside that community. The map was then further enriched by assigning colors to cell towers that represented community membership, he added. All of these data were used to map the strongest networks of connections in the country, Smith continued. Nairobi is the hub of all travel in Kenya and occupies a central role in the map, he said, noting that big cities tend to structure the way people move around the country. He added that there are smaller hubs of travel in the country, such as Lake Victoria, central areas north of Nairobi, and along the coast between Nairobi and Mombasa. Smith described how the investigators used the data to compare the ways that people were moving around with the ways that people were moving parasites around the country, by identifying *sources*—places where people tend to come from—and *sinks*—places where people tend to go. He explained that they created a color-coded human travel map to compare to the known malaria parasite sources and sinks across the country.

Smith reported that after analyzing the maps, the macroscopic-level picture showed virtually no malaria transmission in Nairobi; that is, there were many parasites moving into the city, but not moving out of the city to the rest of the country. He said one reason Nairobi is a popular city to live is because it does not play a dominant role in malaria transmission, compared to Lake Victoria, which is a source of malaria transmission that exports malaria to the rest of Kenya. Smith explained that malaria moves in two ways: people visiting endemic areas may become infected during their

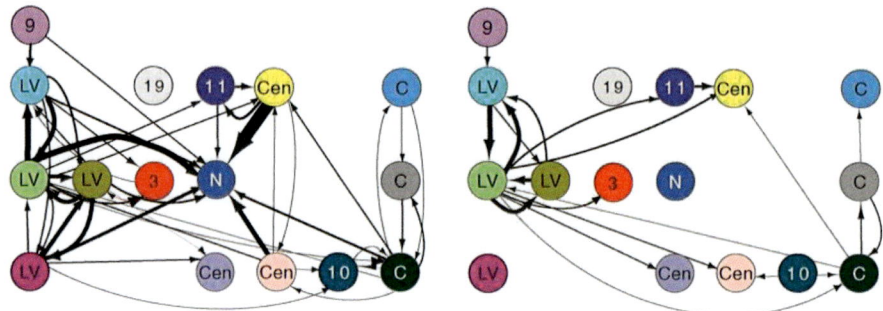

FIGURE 3-3 Travel networks of humans and parasites between settlements and regions in Kenya.
Left: Average monthly parasite importation by returning residents, by region.
Right: Average monthly parasite importation by visitors.
NOTES: Regions near Lake Victoria (LV), in Nairobi (N), in the central areas (Cen), and along the coast (C) are labeled accordingly. Nodes are numbered and shaded to correspond to 1 of 20 risk regions; however, nodes may share a geographic label but be shaded differently according to risk region. Arrows indicate direction of human or parasite movement from primary settlements to visited settlements.
SOURCES: Smith presentation, December 12, 2017; Wesolowski et al., 2012. From Wesolowski, A., N. Eagle, A. Tatem, D. Smith, A. Noor, R. W. Snow, and C. O. Buckee. 2012. Quantifying the impact of human mobility on malaria. *Science* 338(6104):267–270. Reprinted with permission from the American Association for the Advancement of Science.

stay and carry parasites back to their home, or infected people can carry the parasites with them when they visit other places, which can potentially contribute to onward infection if the destination is receptive to transmission. The investigators calculated a measure of risk using an estimate of the proportion of people who are infected, he added, as well as a measure of the number of people traveling from Nairobi, getting infected, and bringing it home. He used Figure 3-3 to illustrate how Nairobi imports malaria from many different places, particularly the areas around Lake Victoria (Figure 3-3 left); however, people traveling to Nairobi are not being infected at all (Figure 3-3 right). According to Smith, the predominant reason for these findings is that Nairobi does not have many anopheline mosquitos, the vector for malaria, for ecological reasons. He added that Nairobi has had anopheline vectors in the past as evidenced by massive malaria epidemics at the end of the previous century, so transmission is possible in Nairobi.

Shifting Vector Transmission in the Built Environment

Smith explained that there are global patterns of shifting vector transmission in urban built environments. He cited Nairobi as an example of how some vector species tend to decline and disappear from urban centers, while others thrive in the same settings. Malaria prevalence tends to be much lower in urban centers, he noted. This is because of a global pattern in which cities tend to lose their anopheline vectors as they develop, he explained, but the anophelines tend to get replaced by *Aedes aegypti* mosquitos that can thrive in urban centers. This catalyzes a shift in the built environment away from malaria and toward dengue and arboviral transmission, which is a mounting problem in urban centers around the world. This known pattern is one of the reasons why Nairobi was immediately put on alert when Mombasa had a dengue fever outbreak, he noted. He added that this type of shift has been documented in Ecuador (Cifuentes et al., 2013).

He reported that the country saw a massive decline in malaria cases between 2001 and 2010 overall, but there was an uptick in dengue cases over the same period (he also noted that dengue did not exist in Ecuador until around 1997). As part of the malaria mapping project in Kenya, he added, the investigators analyzed mosquito-borne pathogen transmission by plotting the ratio of observed clinical cases to estimated imported infections in the city (Wesolowski et al., 2012). They found that transmission was not occurring in Kibera, one of the biggest and most well-known slums in the city, but it was occurring in the wealthier neighborhoods and suburbs where people have large green spaces and yards.

DISCUSSION

The discussion opened with Jennifer Gardy, assistant professor in the School of Population and Public Health, University of British Columbia, asking if there are slums in high-income countries, for example, in settings like a refugee camp in Calais or in Canada's First Nations communities, such as Attawapiskat. Riley explained that it depends on which elements of the definition of slums are applied. According to the UN definition, the largest slum in the United States is located in Los Angeles, he said, and there are other communities in the United States as well as Canada and European countries that would meet certain elements of the definition of a slum. He also noted that Brazil is now considered an upper middle-income country.

Peter Daszak, president of EcoHealth Alliance, asked how slums fit into the changing patterns of cities at the macro level. Smith remarked that in the early 1980s the Guasmo Sur barrio in Guayaquil, Ecuador, was considered the biggest slum in the world, formed by poor residents squatting in the area and siphoning power from existing lines. Initially, the city governance tried to raze the area but then relented, he explained, and within 4 years, they had provided an infrastructure including roads, sewage, drainage, and metered electricity. He said that this type of transition and development can happen quickly if governments are incentivized, and it can help to mitigate infectious disease transmission.

Daszak also asked whether it would be useful to intensify research efforts for looking at fomite risks, air circulation, and pathogen transmission in slums. Li replied that there are research opportunities focusing on slums with the potential to help many people. For example, he said there have been proposals to study carbon dioxide measurements in buildings to see what is happening to the air. He added that lack of access to water for hand washing has been studied in the context of children under 5 years of age contracting respiratory infections in their homes. Riley added that he collaborates with people who do this type of work in slums, such as one researcher who studies indoor air pollution caused by cooking with biofuels in rural areas and now is applying this work to slums, but more researchers are needed. Research is currently focused on environmental exposure issues, he noted, but emphasized that it is ultimately the pathogens that determine the health outcomes. Therefore, research efforts should be focused on both issues, he added.

David Nabarro, advisor on health and sustainability at 4SD, asked three questions about studies that examine health outcomes in urban and slum settings. He first asked whether there have been comparative studies of incidence rates for specific diseases in different urban settings. Riley said that such studies are challenging to do, but he has used the health metrics, such as disability-adjusted life years (DALYs), to assess the burden of disease, particularly TB, in Rio de Janeiro. In the last census, he explained, Brazil used the UN's definition of slums to categorize different neighborhoods as slums or nonslums, which was used to examine the relative burdens of TB. They found differences in the DALY gap, which they categorized according to gender characteristics, electricity provision in the communities, water services, sewage services, and others. This enabled them to understand with greater granularity how this disease contributes to different types of neighborhoods in the same city. He suggested that this is preferable to looking at incidence, because DALYs allow the quality of life in these communities to be quantified. However, he noted that there are not many similar studies, because they require a census to categorize communities as slums or nonslums.

Nabarro's second question was if studies have examined the seasonality of disease incidence in the same urban setting at different times of the year. Riley replied that, although there are known seasonal patterns to different diseases, they have not yet studied seasonality of disease incidence in urban settings like Rio de Janeiro. Li reported that seasonality for influenza is being studied. He explained that seasonality involves atmospheric conditions, temperature, and humidity and surmised that indoor conditions likely determine some of those factors in the urban built environment, where people spend much of their time indoors. He added that for influenza there are good data on outdoor conditions from weather monitoring stations that constantly provide data, but indoor environments are so diversified that the data are not readily available. Smith added that malaria is associated with rainfall and temperature, and it has migration-driven patterns as well as patterns driven by seasonal transmission. In Nairobi, for example, there is an uptick in malaria cases right after Christmas when people return to the city after time at home for the holidays. The pattern of seasonal migration is also a factor, he said, as people abandon their farms and move into cities to work, bringing malaria with them (see Chapter 4 for a discussion on seasonality of leptospirosis in Brazil).

Nabarro's third question was if any studies have linked occupations of slum residents, such as rubbish picking, to health outcomes. Riley said that occupation contributes to different types of health outcomes, such as in Brazil, where leptospirosis is highly prevalent and certainly associated with occupation in some slums. For example, he said that males tend to have higher incidence of leptospirosis, probably because they spend more time outside in occupations involving exposure to contaminated bodies of water. Riley added that interpersonal injuries are major contributors to health outcomes, noting that his studies comparing TB burden in slum and nonslum communities found that the DALY gap was reversed among young adult males in Rio de Janeiro (that is, the DALY was higher among the nonslum community young adult males) (Marlow et al., 2015). He explained this unexpected reversal, despite one-quarter of all TB DALYS being associated with slum conditions, by noting that many who are incarcerated or dead due to interpersonal violence are plausibly young adult males who live in slums, and their information was not available. He said that this type of analysis can help assess what is happening on the ground in these communities beyond just infectious diseases. Li said there are data available about occupational transmission of community-acquired methicillin-resistant *Staphylococcus aureus*. In Hong Kong, he reported, the data show that infection rates among the estimated 200,000 to 300,000 domestic helpers in the city are quite high compared to the general community (CHP, 2007; Government of Hong Kong, 2017). In cities where foreign domestic helpers tend to do much of the housework, he said, it would be helpful to investigate infection and transmission among people who work in that sector.

Mary Wilson, clinical professor of epidemiology and biostatistics at the University of California, San Francisco, noted that during outbreaks of respiratory infections studies have identified superspreaders who are responsible for transmitting a large number of cases; she asked whether host factors, environmental conditions, or other circumstances are associated with superspreaders. Li replied that he studied superspreaders of SARS and observed that, in some outbreaks, the environment magnified the sources.

One of his studies analyzed the superspreading events in Singapore and Hong Kong and found that, compared to Singapore, each event in Hong Kong produced a number of infections that was an order of magnitude greater (Li et al., 2004). He noted that it is difficult to tell whether such events are because of host factors, index patients, or density of people and buildings. He added that another event occurred during the 2015 outbreak of Middle East respiratory syndrome in Seoul, Korea, when engineers neglected to install the air supply in a particular hospital room (see Chapter 4 discussion for more on the issue of superspreaders).

Eva Harris, professor of infectious diseases and director of the Center for Global Public Health at the University of California, Berkeley, commented that emerging data from Brazil and other places suggest that socioeconomic status has a large effect on microcephaly outcomes. This may be caused by such sociological factors as access to abortion, she posited, or it might be affected by other factors such as nutrition and its effect on an individual's immune system, microbiome, and disease outcomes. Harris suggested trying to identify direct risk factors and better understand how those factors can work through the biology and the immunology to the disease outcome. Gardy suggested looking at the intergenerational effects of slums on health to consider the developmental origins of health and disease as well as how impacts on maternal health propagate to subsequent generations. For example, she suggested looking at the sequelae of children who were not raised in slums but whose parents were raised in slum environments.

Edward You, supervisory special agent in the Federal Bureau of Investigation's Weapons of Mass Destruction Directorate, raised the issue of modern urbanization contributing to an increasingly controlled environment in which people are more immunologically naïve, which, in turn, drives increased incidence of diseases like obesity and asthma. While the focus is often on disease transmission and pathogens perturbing the system, he wondered whether the controlled environment may also be setting populations up for failure in the future. Riley noted an increase in obesity in slum communities in India and Brazil that is likely caused by changes in nutrition, including overnutrition. He said that the use of antibiotics and exposure to antibiotics in the environment, food, and water have altered the physiology of people's bodies—such as the intestinal microbiota—in ways that contribute to diabetes and thus lead to various infectious disease health outcomes. Riley suggested studying mechanisms that influence people's immune systems, such as the modernization of food habits, the globalization of the food trade, and the consequential changes in behavioral health and eating behavior.

Lonnie King, professor and dean emeritus at The Ohio State University College of Veterinary Medicine, remarked that food needs increase as the number of people in slums and urban areas increases in real numbers. He noted that the structure of agriculture and food production is changing and moving closer as people move into urban settings, but workers are still moving back and forth between agricultural communities and cities. King suggested that this gives rise to concern about zoonotic diseases as well as foodborne illnesses.

Marcos Espinal, director of communicable diseases and health analysis at the Pan American Health Organization, asked Riley about his call for action now instead of waiting for the SDGs. He asked if there are any proposals beyond UN-Habitat's conclusion after its conference in 2016 that the current urbanization model is costly and unsustainable, and a new agenda is needed to upgrade slum communities and address systemic issues that extend beyond health. Thomas Scott, distinguished professor in the Department of Entomology and Nematology at the University of California, Davis, added that the SDGs' longer-term solutions are not mutually exclusive with immediate actions to improve housing, sanitation, and water supplies; he suggested finding ways to integrate both types of strategies. Riley said that the SDGs are valuable guidelines, and he is not denigrating their importance, but there are issues that need immediate action. He used the analogy of a person hit by a car: the immediate response is to help the victim, but long-term efforts should help prevent those types of accidents from occurring at all. Both types of activities are necessary, he suggested.

Dominguez-Bello posited an optimistic perspective and imagined that, in a century or two from now, the world will have at least partially solved the problem of inequities and improved the slums. But at the same time, she imagined, people will be living in crowded urban centers, while urban farms and agriculture produce food, and the human microbiome will be degraded with urbanization. She asked if urban planners and architects should be responsible for predicting and intervening against future microbial diseases in cities. Riley said he has a dark vision of the future and predicted that the issues faced by urban slums will get much worse before they improve; he said that the effect of slums on global health will be evident long before the effects of climate change and did not envision any concrete, immediate solutions. Li took a more optimistic stance, predicting that humans will be smart enough to find those solutions and create better urban centers. Smith said that his process-based perspective is focused on understanding how slums are created, how they persist, and how they go away. He predicted that those processes would not change, and there will still be slums, even if they are different types of slums.

Nabarro said that some have argued that living in an urban slum is better than living in a bad rural existence. With climate change affecting production potential in so many parts of the world, he said, movement to cities will likely increase, and slums will serve as a refuge and haven for people who are escaping real poverty in rural areas. Riley contended that urban slum populations actually fare much worse than the rural poor. He said that poverty is not necessarily related to slums, because slums have a distinct set of conditions and health outcomes. He added that aggregate data suggesting that people living in urban settings are better off are based on comparisons that are not apt. Peter Sands, executive director designate for The Global Fund to Fight AIDS, Tuberculosis and Malaria, cautioned against disaggregating urban statistics to separate slum data without disaggregating the rural statistics, because people who move to urban slums may originate from the worst parts of the rural area.

Nabarro suggested that the alternative to hoping for a future without slums is to collectively plan for the influx of people who will move to cities in search of work and opportunities. He suggested finding ways to improve slum conditions for those people, when there is often government resistance to improving infrastructure and living conditions in slums that is premised on keeping people living there from becoming permanent residents. Sands asked if there are any good models for low-cost ways to absorb large numbers of relatively poor people into a dense urban environment. Riley replied that only time will tell the effect of existing models because progress can be undercut by unpredictable political and economic circumstances—in Brazil, for example, poverty was greatly reduced during former President Lula's tenure (2003 to 2011), but those programs are currently being rolled back, and the positive trends are reversing. Riley also cautioned that all slum communities are different, even within the same city or large slum area, and a model that works in one place may not necessarily work in another. Christopher Dye, director of strategy, policy, and information at the Office of the Director-General of WHO, remarked that there is a great deal of knowledge about what does work. For example, he explained that the Lula era contributed to a better understanding of the effectiveness of initiatives, such as community-based health insurance and cash transfer schemes. He said that the challenge is to take that knowledge of initiatives that work and implement them.

4

Translating Conceptual Models of Infectious Disease Transmission and Control into Practice

The second half of session 1 featured case studies for translating conceptual models of infectious disease control and transmission into practice. The session was moderated by Marcos Espinal, director of communicable diseases and health analysis at the Pan American Health Organization. Frank Mahoney, senior immunization officer at the International Federation of Red Cross and Red Crescent Societies, described the effect the West Africa Ebola virus disease (EVD) outbreak had on the epidemiology of other infectious diseases. Emily Gurley, associate scientist in the Department of Epidemiology at the Johns Hopkins Bloomberg School of Public Health, described efforts to control the transmission of waterborne diseases in Dhaka, Bangladesh. Albert Ko, professor and chair of the Department of Epidemiology of Microbial Diseases at the Yale School of Public Health, examined the transmission and control of leptospirosis and Zika virus in Brazilian slums. Robin Wood, chief executive officer of the Desmond Tutu HIV Centre and Foundation at the University of Cape Town, explored transmission and control of tuberculosis (TB) in Cape Town, South Africa.

EFFECT OF THE WEST AFRICA EBOLA VIRUS DISEASE OUTBREAK ON OTHER INFECTIOUS DISEASES

Frank Mahoney, senior immunization officer at the International Federation of Red Cross and Red Crescent Societies, spoke about the effect of the West Africa EVD outbreak on the epidemiology of other infectious diseases based on his experience as a medical epidemiologist with the U.S.

Centers for Disease Control and Prevention (CDC) during the epidemic. He began his presentation by sharing the case of diplomat Patrick Sawyer who was being monitored in Monrovia, Liberia, for suspected EVD in July 2014. Sawyer left the country and traveled to Lagos, Nigeria, where he was admitted to a local hospital with a provisional diagnosis of malaria. The chief medical officer at the hospital suspected EVD, and the diagnosis was confirmed 2 days before Sawyer died. Mahoney reported that 72 health care workers and airport staff overall were exposed to the disease through Sawyer. To illustrate how the exposure occurred, he cited a statement from the case investigation form made by a health care worker who cared for Sawyer:

> On getting to the patient, I discovered his intravenous line was by his side and picked it up with bare hands to hang on the drip stand. I called the nurse to assist the patient to [the] toilet. I had a cut on my hand and did not remember to wash my hands until much later in the shift.

At the time, he said, many health care workers in the area were not trained to scrupulously reduce exposure to infectious bodily fluids.

Effect of the Outbreak on the Health Workforce and Health Services Provision

According to Mahoney, the EVD outbreak in West Africa had a substantial effect on the health systems in the region between 2014 and 2015, affecting both the health workforce and the provision of health services in the region. During the epidemic, he said, a total of 815 health care workers were infected, and of the known outcomes, the mortality rate was 66 percent (WHO, 2015). Early in the outbreak, he reported, a high proportion of the EVD cases occurred among the health workforce (see Figure 4-1). However, training on infection control for every health worker helped to reduce the proportion of health care worker deaths to around 1 percent by the end of the outbreak (WHO, 2015). The geographic distribution of EVD infection among health care workers in West Africa spanned both urban and rural settings, noted Mahoney. A diverse range of health care workers were infected, he said, mainly workers who had primary contact with patients, such as nurses and nurse aids. He explained that this had a major effect on the health care system, such as limiting the provision of services, closing many facilities, and raising concerns among the health care workers about becoming infected in health care settings—especially when managing patients with febrile illness and/or hemorrhage. At the community level, he said that people also had fears of becoming infected by receiving treatment

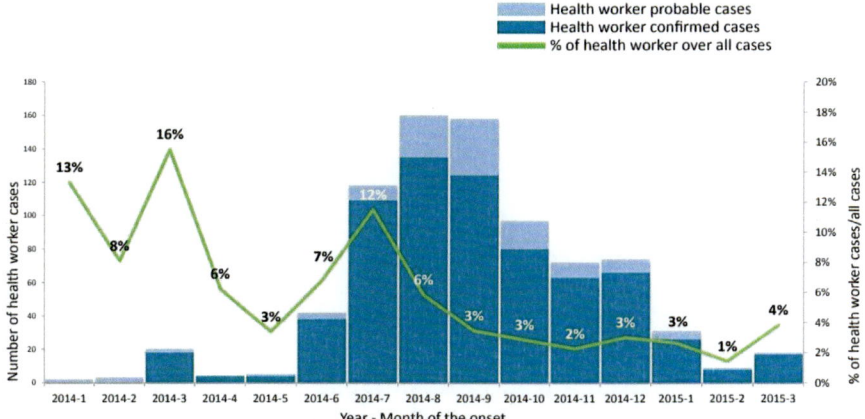

FIGURE 4-1 Number of probable and confirmed Ebola virus disease (EVD) infections among health care workers in Guinea, Liberia, and Sierra Leone (January 2014 to March 2015).
NOTE: All cases include health worker and nonhealth worker confirmed and probable cases.
SOURCES: Mahoney presentation, December 12, 2017; WHO, 2015. Reprinted from *Health worker Ebola infections in Guinea, Liberia, and Sierra Leone, preliminary report*, page 3, Copyright (2015).

in health care settings and would tend to seek care from community health care workers.

Mahoney reported that there was a subsequent decrease in the use of health care services during the outbreak, which has been documented by multiple studies on the effect of the EVD outbreak on health care delivery in West Africa. For example, he cited a study that investigated the average monthly consultations for children under 5 years of age before and during the EVD outbreak in Sierra Leone, finding reductions in visits for malaria (–27 percent), acute respiratory infection or pneumonia (–27 percent), and acute watery diarrhea (–38 percent); however, there was an 80 percent increase in the number of patients who came in with measles (Sesay et al., 2017). He also described a community-level, population-based survey assessing health care use during and after the EVD outbreak in Liberia, which found that in December 2014 (around the peak of the outbreak), among the 25 percent of households reporting a sick child in the previous 2 weeks, only 40 percent of them sought care for the sick children in the health care system; this rebounded to between 80 and 90 percent by March 2015 (Morse et al., 2016). During the peak of the epidemic, people stopped accessing care, he said, but it seemed that they quickly recovered. He cited several more studies documenting the negative effects of EVD on health care delivery in the region:

- In hospitals and public health clinics in Guinea, there were decreases in HIV testing, in Pentavalent 1 and 3 vaccinations, and in visits for acute respiratory infections and acute watery diarrhea (Barden-O'Fallon et al., 2015).
- Across 15 facilities in Sierra Leone, there was a decrease in outpatient visits (Elston et al., 2016).
- In a hospital setting in Guinea, there were decreases in clinic or pharmacy visits and in antiretroviral compliance (Cisse et al., 2015).
- In mobile treatment facilities in Guinea, there were decreases in outpatient visits (–40 percent), in HIV testing (–46 percent), in enrollment in HIV care (–47 percent), and in new diagnoses of HIV (–53 percent) (Leuenberger et al., 2015).

Changes in the Epidemiology of Priority Diseases

Mahoney explained that changes in health care use caused by the EVD outbreak in West Africa gave rise to concerns about changes in the epidemiology of priority diseases in the region—HIV, malaria, and TB. He described a study that modeled the effect of the EVD outbreak on the malaria, HIV, and TB disease burdens in Guinea, Liberia, and Sierra Leone. He said that the analysis attributed approximately 7,000 additional deaths from malaria as a result of the outbreak and a change of approximately 50 percent in malaria-attributable mortality rates in all three countries.[1] For HIV, he said, they estimated around 1,000 additional deaths and a change in the HIV-attributable mortality rate of around 15 percent.[2] He added that for TB they estimated around 3,000 additional deaths and a subsequent 50 to 60 percent change in the TB-attributable mortality rate (Parpia et al., 2016).[3] He described a different study that found increases in untreated malaria cases of 45 percent in Guinea, 88 percent in Sierra Leone, and 140 percent in Liberia in 2014; researchers estimated the disease burden at 3.5 million additional untreated cases and 10,900 additional malaria-attributable deaths (Walker et al., 2015).

Other diseases were affected as well, noted Mahoney. People stopped

---

[1] Based on an estimated 50 percent reduction in treatment coverage among children less than 5 years of age.

[2] Based on 50 percent reduction in antiretroviral coverage among persons 15 to 49 years of age.

[3] Based on 50 percent reduction in treatment coverage for both drug-susceptible and drug-resistant TB.

coming for their immunizations, he said, and Guinea, Liberia, and Sierra Leone all experienced reductions in coverage for both diphtheria-tetanus-pertussis and measles, leading to an increase in susceptibility, based on World Health Organization (WHO)-United Nations Children's Fund (UNICEF) estimates of vaccination coverage. According to 2015 estimates, he reported, there were large numbers of children up to 3 years of age in Liberia who were susceptible to measles, and as expected, all of the countries experienced measles outbreaks in 2015; he noted that they all implemented measles supplemental immunization campaigns to mitigate those outbreaks. He described another study on all-cause mortality in Moyamba District, Sierra Leone, which reviewed burial team data for a 5-month period (November 2014 to April 2015). He said they reported 496 deaths among children less than 1 year of age, 786 among children less than 5 years of age, and around 1,300 deaths among persons less than 50 years of age. He noted that Ebola caused only 2 percent of these deaths and that mortality was 3.4 times higher than the average mortality in the preceding 3 years. Although death registration may not be entirely accurate, he added, it still represents a threefold increase (Elston et al., 2016).

Mahoney reiterated that the EVD outbreak had major effects on the health workforce and on health service delivery in the region, which led to decreases in access and use of services for major infectious diseases. He noted that models predicted an increase in subsequent mortality that was difficult to measure in practice, with only limited data showing resulting increases in mortality. However, he suggested that local measures may have mitigated this effect, such as interventions against measles and mass drug administration for malaria.

Management of Outbreaks in Urban Settings

Mahoney discussed some potential lessons that might be gleaned from the management of the EVD outbreak in West Africa, using specific examples from the outbreak management in Liberia and in Nigeria. He related that early in the outbreak in Liberia—when the number of suspect cases was doubling every 2 weeks—a presidential task force was deployed to manage the situation. He explained that the task force implemented quarantine in West Point, the largest slum in the capital of Liberia, which led to conflict with and resistance from the community. He said that it ultimately created mistrust in the government regarding the whole epidemic response. Providers participating in the response were also concerned, he added, as Montserrado County was overwhelmed with cases: there were not enough Ebola treatment unit (ETU) beds, people were dying in the streets, and models were predicting hundreds of thousands of EVD cases. Responders debated about the type of care that should be provided (ETU model of care, home care, or transit centers), he said, and they were concerned about managing patients within a health care system that had already been hugely affected by the beginning of the outbreak.

To develop a Liberian strategy, Mahoney said meetings were convened with international partners in August 2014. He said the key elements of the strategy were early identification and isolation of suspect patients (through intensified surveillance, contact tracing, and clinical management in dedicated treatment centers); safe transportation; prevention of transmission in the health care setting; and safe burials. He noted that the strategy did not include treatment within the existing health care system, distribution of home health care kits, wide-scale support for water and distribution of hygiene kits, or the involuntary quarantine of infected households.

Mahoney presented a range of challenges related to the construction of ETUs in Liberia. He said they are costly, in terms of both money and human resources, because 400 health care workers were required per 100-bed ETU, and few support organizations had the relevant experience. One strategy for addressing these challenges, he said, was to set up an ETU in an abandoned hospital. He explained that the Island Clinic in Montserrado County, Liberia, was renovated into a 100-bed hospital with WHO support and was managed by the government. He reported that it was filled within hours of opening and had more than 200 admissions in the first week, but within 2 months of opening in 2014, there was a remarkable drop in admissions in Montserrado County (WHO, 2014). He reported that Nigeria also experienced a crisis when faced with several highly probable cases of EVD but had nowhere to care for them. He explained that they resolved this by setting up an ETU in an abandoned hospital ward in Lagos, where they set up improvised hygiene stations and clinical staff were mentored by people with previous ETU experience (Shuaib et al., 2014).

After the initial decline of EVD cases in more populated areas, Mahoney said they faced rural outbreaks of EVD in isolated communities in Liberia caused by infected people leaving the city and seeding outbreaks in these areas. He explained that the response to those rural outbreaks was called the Rapid Isolation and Treatment of Ebola strategy, which served as a complement to the other outbreak response activities. Over time, he said, the strategy helped reduce the intervention period interval quite substantially over the course of the epidemic. Mahoney concluded by suggesting the following set of strategies for maintaining the capacity for preparedness moving forward:

- Rapidly detect and isolate patients.
- Identify—in advance—facilities to manage patients with hemorrhagic fever.
- Embed infection control practices into everyday practice.

- Maintain skills of clinical staff.
- Engage with communities for effective management of response.

WATERBORNE DISEASES IN DHAKA, BANGLADESH

Emily Gurley, associate scientist in the Department of Epidemiology at the Johns Hopkins Bloomberg School of Public Health, gave a presentation on the waterborne transmission of cholera in the urban built environment, illustrating practical strategies for preventing and mitigating the transmission of cholera that have been used in Dhaka, Bangladesh. She opened by lamenting that, from an epidemiological perspective, not enough progress has been made since John Snow's seminal work tracing the 1854 cholera epidemic in London to the Broad Street pump by mapping the hotspots of disease. She noted that many current strategies for cholera remain similar to Snow's work. Gurley said that progress has been made in many other ways, however. For example, she reported that Millennium Development Goal (MDG) 7c, which aimed to halve the population without sustainable access to safe drinking water, was achieved through collaborative efforts and commitment to the goal. That said, she noted that achieving sustainability of access and safety of drinking water remains a struggle—not only in how to go about it but how to measure it. For the purposes of the MDGs, she noted, sustainable access to safe water was defined as the proportion of the population using *improved* drinking water sources. She explained that improved sources are designed and constructed to deliver safe water, such as covered sources that are expected to be protected from microbial contamination (for example, this would not include a lake or an open shallow well).

Gurley reported that worldwide there is still a large degree of heterogeneity and inequity in terms of access to safe drinking water. In many countries, she said, the situation may appear relatively good, but within a country's political boundaries, there is often substantial heterogeneity in access to safe water. She explained that this is the case in Bangladesh, where WHO data estimate that between 76 and 85 percent of the population have been using improved drinking water sources since 2000, but there are reasons to be skeptical that this trend is reflected countrywide (WHO, 2017c).

Reducing Cholera Transmission in Arichpur of Dhaka, Bangladesh

Since 2009, Gurley has been working on reducing waterborne infections in Arichpur of Tongi Township in Dhaka, Bangladesh. She explained that Arichpur is densely populated, with around 50,000 residents in an area of roughly one-half of a square kilometer. She added that the community has few high-rise buildings, but adjacent to the community is a large open campground where 5 million people converge from Bangladesh and 150 countries every January for Bishwa Ijtema, the largest gathering of Muslims in the world. Gurley explained that Arichpur is a very wet place, bounded to the south by a river and subject to monsoon floods; the drainage is poor and streets are prone to flooding, which makes them difficult to navigate.

Despite its wet climate, Gurley noted, it is difficult to access safe drinking water in Arichpur. She noted that Bangladesh has done much work to improve access to drinking water: cities have improved their water sources and the majority of the country's residents have access to improved water sources, mostly from municipal water supplies (57 percent) (Gurley et al., 2014). However, she said that the safety of those municipal water supplies is uncertain because they are relatively old, and the population has grown faster than the supply and infrastructure can keep up with. She said that many people resort to finding the main water line and creating their own access. She explained that open sewers running through the streets often contain makeshift hoses that run the municipal water supply into homes. She said that this creates many opportunities for contamination, such as breaches in the municipal water lines. She was initially called to work in Arichpur because of an outbreak of hepatitis E caused by a mass contamination of the municipal water supply, which spread quickly through the community and infected around 4,000 people (Gurley et al., 2014).

Gurley explained that they began considering how to address cholera in Arichpur and how to better understand the drivers of the established cholera risk. Understanding those drivers, she said, requires strategies to improve surveillance and to predict the areas and populations that are at the highest risk in the community. She explained that the current standard of cholera surveillance is to wait for people to visit a health facility and be diagnosed, at which point they are usually quite ill already. She deemed this strategy unsatisfactory for multiple reasons. She said that it identifies only severe cases, especially in areas with poor access to care. She added that it is not timely, because by the time severe cases present themselves, it is likely that a number of other cases in the community already occurred, and the opportunity to prevent the outbreak may have been lost. To improve their strategy, she said, they aimed to build a cholera surveillance system that would ideally be able to identify the etiologies—including being able to find mild and severe cases to study—and would enable notification as close to the time of infection as possible. They carried out studies on three potential surveillance strategies: cholera prediction through pharmacy sales; the Choleraphone community surveillance intervention; and cluster analysis of cholera risk factors in the community.

Cholera Prediction Through Pharmacy Sales

Gurley described the first study, where she and her colleagues decided to try a cholera surveillance strategy using data on sales of oral rehydration solution (ORS) among pharmacies and drug sellers as an early warning system for cholera. In a survey study, she said, they enrolled 50 of the 120 drug sellers identified in Arichpur and asked them to send the researchers a daily text message with the number of ORS packets sold at the end of the day. She explained that the ORS sales data were compared to the traditional cholera surveillance system that was already in place in Dhaka. The study found that between April and October 2013, cholera cases represented about 22 percent of total diarrhea hospitalizations, she reported, and analysis revealed seasonality to ORS sales that corresponded with the seasonality of diarrhea and cholera (Azman et al., 2015). It also revealed the spatial distribution of cholera sales, she added, when they aligned all the pharmacies based on their locations in the community and found spatial heterogeneity in where the ORS packets were being sold. She said that this spatial heterogeneity also corresponded with where they found cases of diarrhea and cholera. Although they found significant correlations between ORS sales and cholera, she noted, it was not a great predictor because it was only able to provide an early signal 1 day ahead of the cholera. Furthermore, she noted that the data are noisy and not specific enough because ORS interventions in Bangladesh have been so successful that the packets are readily available and commonly used for reasons other than diarrhea treatment.

Choleraphone Surveillance Intervention

Gurley continued to describe another approach in the same community using a surveillance intervention called Choleraphone. They enrolled a cohort of 400 households nested within a study on access to water, she said, and each household was provided with a phone that was recharged every month. Households were asked to call the study team when someone in the house had diarrhea, she explained, and then a health care worker would visit that home to provide ORS and request that the person self-collect a rectal swab. The incidence of diarrhea found through the Choleraphone was compared to a household survey, but she hoped that this approach would provide the etiology and offer a real-time picture of cholera in the community. She said that people did report diarrhea over the phone, but overall the incidence was much lower than expected. She noted that the study population is highly mobile and difficult to study; many enrolled households dropped out for various reasons, such as leaving or moving elsewhere in the community or reluctance to self-collect a rectal swab.

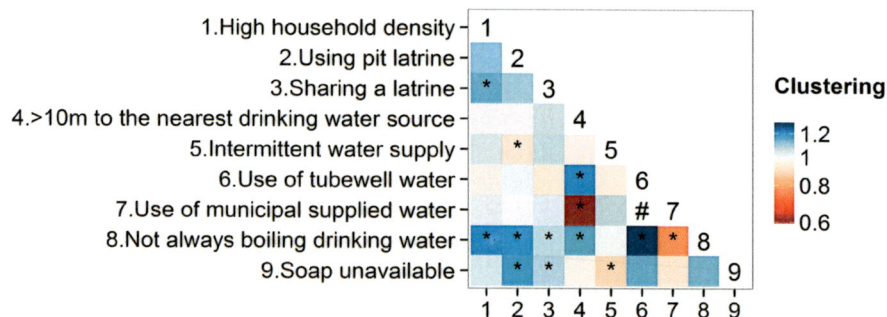

FIGURE 4-2 Co-occurrence of different household-level exposures of high-risk factors for cholera in spatially matched households (matched-sets).
NOTES: Shading of cells indicates estimates of co-occurrence of different exposures and denotes intraclass correlation coefficient estimates between 0.6 and 1.2. Values above 1 suggest a tendency for two exposures to appear in the same households or matched-set closer to each other (co-occurrence of two exposures). Values less than 1 suggest a tendency for two exposures not to appear together. Numbers on the x-axis refer to the corresponding number listed as the high-risk factors for cholera on the y-axis.
* Statistically significant estimates based on 1,000 bootstrap iterations.
# Result not shown because the "Use of municipal supplied water" risk factor was structurally correlated to the "Use of tubewell water" risk factor.
SOURCES: Gurley presentation, December 12, 2017; Bi et al., 2016.

Cluster Analysis of Cholera Risk Factors in the Community

Gurley explained that the third strategy was a study looking at clustering of risk factors for cholera within the community (Bi et al., 2016). For every confirmed case, she explained, they enrolled sets of spatially matched control households and then compared households distributed throughout these communities, looking for spatial clustering of high-risk factors for waterborne disease in general and cholera in particular. She reported that they found a large amount of clustering (see Figure 4-2); for example, households without hand soap were highly clustered with those using pit latrines. Spatially, those risk factors were clustered together within households, she noted, and added that even within this area of high risk, there were pockets that were at much higher risk than others based on what is known about transmission.

Gurley concluded by suggesting that it is useful to appreciate and understand these types of substantial and important spatial heterogeneities in risk, even within a single community, because those clusters of exposure can be targeted for interventions, such as vaccination. She noted that, although good vaccines are available, the ability to deploy them well and in a timely way is an ongoing struggle. They are considering carrying out seroprevalence surveys that could identify where people have been infected previously and help think about risk going forward, she added.

She also suggested that creative, context-specific surveillance solutions are useful. For example, she said that they are interested in looking at intravenous fluids provided by drug sellers when people are feeling particularly sick. Finally, she noted an ongoing struggle to sustain the gains in improved water source access over time. She explained that reduced exposure creates new outbreak opportunities because it reduces the population-level risk of some of these diseases, which creates large pools of susceptible people. In this scenario, breaches and contamination in municipal water supplies and other water sources will likely cause even larger outbreaks than those seen now in places like Dhaka, where people are regularly exposed to those diseases.

EMERGING VECTOR-BORNE AND ZOONOTIC DISEASES IN BRAZILIAN SLUMS

Albert Ko, professor and chair of the Department of Epidemiology of Microbial Diseases at the Yale School of Public Health, discussed emerging vector-borne and zoonotic diseases in Brazilian slum communities. He described some of the challenges related to identifying drivers of transmission in urban slum environments and highlighted the contribution of gradients to disease risk, both between seemingly disparate communities in the urban macroenvironment as well as the slum microenvironment within communities.

Bottlenecks to Spillover Transmission

Providing another conceptual model that was translated into practice, Ko presented a model of bottlenecks to spillover transmission that facilitate or constrain transmission of different diseases between species (Plowright et al., 2017) (see Figure 4-3). He explained that the model traces the bottlenecks through the following path: reservoir distribution, reservoir density, pathogen prevalence, infection intensity, pathogen release, pathogen survival and spread in environmental reservoirs, human exposure, and finally within-host barriers. He said these bottlenecks pose challenges to identifying drivers of transmission and there are further challenges to identifying drivers of transmission in complex urban slum environments. For

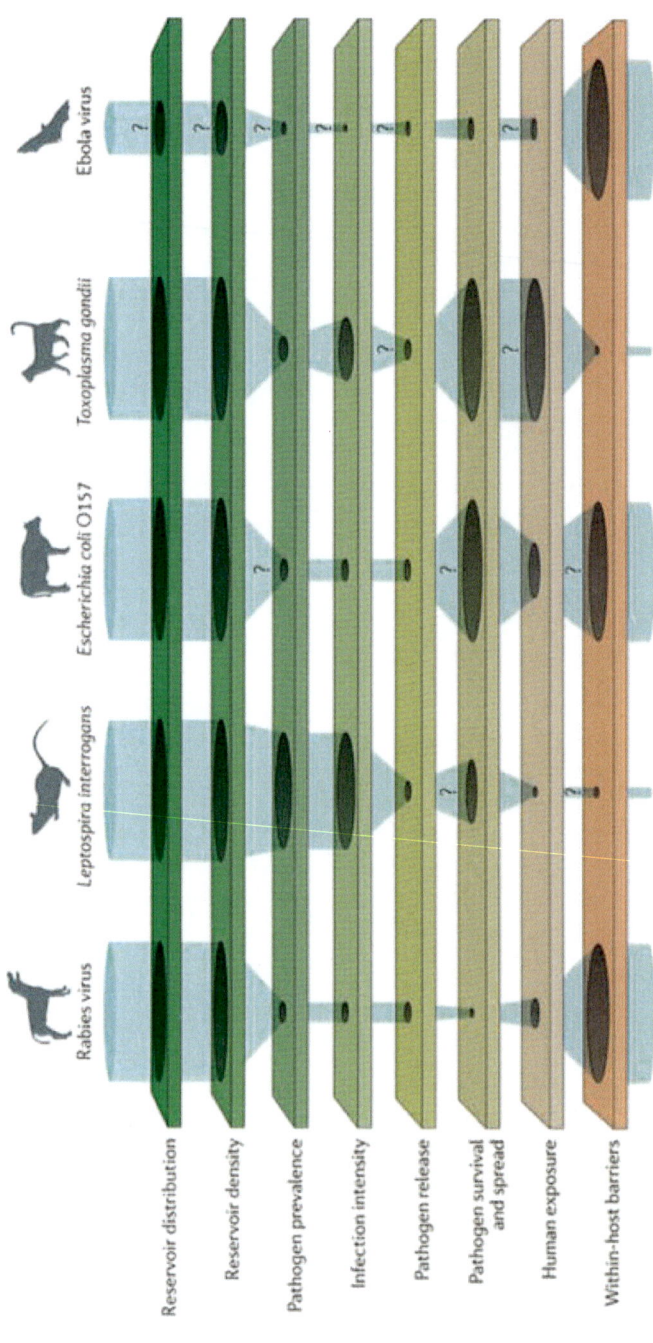

FIGURE 4-3 Different barriers facilitate or constrain the flow of pathogens from one species to another.
NOTES: The width of the gaps between barriers signifies the ease of spillover transmission depending on context. The question marks represent the knowledge gaps in specific pathogens' points of transmission.
SOURCES: Ko presentation, December 12, 2017; Plowright et al., 2017. Reprinted by permission from Springer Customer Service Centre GmbH: Springer Nature. *Nature Reviews Microbiology*. Pathways to zoonotic spillover, Plowright, R. K., C. R. Parrish, H. McCallum, P. J. Hudson, A. I. Ko, A. L. Graham, and J. O. Lloyd-Smith. © 2017.

example, he said, slum environments are not homogeneous communities, but extremely heterogeneous communities. Although heterogeneity can be a challenge, he added, this variation can also provide insight into designing and implementing interventions.

Ko outlined some research challenges related to identifying drivers of transmission. He said that the standard methods for identifying reservoir distributions and reservoir densities are impractical, infeasible, and imprecise. He added that there is a lack of sound environmental sampling methods, particularly for pathogens, and poor linkage between environmental sampling data and human outcomes. He noted that human exposures are highly stochastic processes in urban slum communities, and that researchers must rely on imprecise proxies. Further challenges, according to Ko, are posed by the complex synergisms and the covariation at hand, such as defining the concept of poverty. He believed that a major challenge is that researchers have been limited to modeling static processes rather than dynamic processes because of the difficulty and intensity of the work; as a result, the models exclude dynamic processes of movement or migration including reservoirs, pathogens, and humans.

Release of Bottlenecks: Spillover of Environmentally Transmitted Pathogens

Ko described how the release of bottlenecks leads to the spillover of environmentally transmitted pathogens, including leptospirosis. He explored how ecological changes from urbanization and the growth of slums can contribute to spillover breakthrough via the release of bottlenecks, using the example of work that he and his colleagues have been carrying out in the city of Salvador, Brazil's third largest city at 3 million people. He explained that in Salvador's Pau da Lima periurban slum community, half of the population lives below the poverty line, and because of open sewers and other factors, rats (not humans) are the dominant, biologically successful mammal. He said that rats reside in burrows under earthen stairwells in close proximity to where people live (Cornwall, 2016).

New Epidemiological Pattern of Leptospirosis

Ko said that leptospirosis has emerged as a slum health problem in a new epidemiological pattern that is a consequence of ecological changes juxtaposed with demographic and social changes. He explained that leptospirosis was traditionally a rural-based zoonotic spirochetal disease in which the pathogen (the spirochete) is harbored in the renal tube and shed into the environment, where humans come into contact either directly with the reservoir or indirectly through the environment. He said that under this new epidemiological pattern, which is evident in Salvador and many other major Brazilian urban centers, there are rainfall-associated leptospirosis epidemics that attack the same urban slum communities in a predictable pattern each year. Transmission of leptospirosis in Salvador is primarily rat-borne (primarily *Rattus norvegicus*) and due to a single serovar agent, he said. There are similar conditions of poverty and climate in communities throughout the developing world, he added. In Brazil alone, there are more than 12,000 cases, with high case fatality rates: more than 10 percent for Weil's disease,[4] and more than 50 percent for leptospirosis-associated severe pulmonary hemorrhagic syndrome (Ko et al., 1999; McBride et al., 2005).

The dynamics of rat reservoirs are key drivers of transmission, explained Ko. His team has carried out extensive rat-trapping surveys in Salvador, and has determined that the predominant mode of intraspecific transmission is environmentally mediated. He reported that carriage rates in the rat populations are more than 80 percent, and that each rat sheds approximately 10^{10} bacteria per day (Costa et al., 2015). He said that traditional capture–recapture methods do not work for *Rattus norvegicus* to estimate rat abundance, so they use an inexpensive tracking board method as a proxy for abundance (Hacker et al., 2016). Ceramic tiles painted with lampblack are set out overnight to capture rat paw prints, tail marks, and scratches, which are used toward densely sampling rat abundance. He reported that population abundance and pathogen shedding vary significantly across slum environments, yet the rat-related factors do not vary over season and time.

Rainfall as a Driver for Exposure to the Leptospiral Pathogen

Ko explained that they searched for potential temporal factors or drivers that cause seasonality of leptospirosis epidemics in humans, despite the rat-related factors themselves not appearing to be seasonal. They conducted a 10-year time series analysis of more than 2,000 leptospirosis hospitalizations to generate a fairly robust predictive model, he reported, which is being used in Salvador to identify outbreaks and allocate resources in real time. He said they found that lower temperatures may actually promote pathogen survival in the environment, and subsequently infection risks. They also found that even small amounts of rainfall—not only extreme events—also contribute to risk, he added, with increases in cases (including a lag time of 1 to 2 weeks that is roughly the incubation period for leptospirosis) indicating that exposures occur during or shortly after rainfall events in urban slum communities.

---

[4] Weil's disease occurs when leptospirosis infection in humans causes life-threatening complications, including jaundice, renal dysfunction, and hemorrhaging.

Ko said they conducted a study based on their finding that higher leptospiral pathogen loads are also associated with seasonal periods of heavy rainfall in urban slum communities (Casanovas-Massana et al., 2018). They used longitudinal sampling of open sewage and standing water and used quantitative polymerase chain reaction (qPCR) to detect genome equivalents of leptospirosis, he explained. He reported that high probabilities of quantitative PCR-positive samples and higher loads of leptospirosis were associated with the rainy season, and particularly associated the leptospirosis load or the probability of finding leptospirosis in sewage with the rainy season. He added that morning sampling during the rainy season detected higher loads than in the afternoon—probably because rats tend to be nocturnal, so there is probably more shedding over time in the evenings. The valley bottoms in the community also had higher loads of leptospirosis, he said. He suggested that, based on these findings, open sewers serve as transmission sources of leptospirosis in slum communities. According to Ko, the findings also illustrate the contribution of hydrology and the movement of the pathogen through water, sewage, and soil as potential drivers for leptospirosis during the rain seasons.

Potential Influences of the Environment and Social Gradients on Infection Transmission

Ko described a study that demonstrates the influence of the environment and social gradients on *Leptospira* infection. A long-term cohort study in Pau da Lima used tracking boards and surveys to identify risk factors associated with spillover infections or exposures, he said, and analysis found several significant covariates (Reis et al., 2008). The rat linear predictor (based on tracking board outputs) was significant, he reported, as was the cumulative rainfall experienced by the cohort participants. He said that greater distance to a public trash dump lowered the risk for infection, probably because trash is a food source for rats. He suggested that this finding is an example of a definable infrastructure deficiency that drives transmission. In the context of synergisms and covariation, he reported that the logarithm of household income per capita, which captures both environmental and social factors, was also significantly associated with risk. He said that the poorest land quality is at the bottom of valleys in the slum community, which is consistent with a larger pattern of vulnerable populations within slums residing in areas with the worst land quality.

Ko reported that the social gradient was captured in this study by socioeconomic status, which was associated with risk for leptospirosis. He explained that, for every $1 per capita household income per day, there is a decrease in risk of exposure to leptospirosis. He added that they also found a linear increase in risk among people until they reach 30 years of age, after which it plateaus. He said that males had significantly increased risk, suggesting that adult young males tend to engage in risky behaviors that lead to exposures; for example, he added, after a rainfall people dig out the open sewers to create a barrier so that it does not overflow and flood their households in the next rainfall event.

Ko suggested that disparities in Zika and congenital Zika syndrome outcomes in slum versus nonslum communities in Pau da Lima illustrate the broad effect of inequities related to infectious disease transmission, both within slum communities and between slum and nonslum communities. He said that the Zika epidemic in Pau da Lima is an example of an epidemic that breaks the typical paradigm of focusing on disease rather than process. He reported that seroincidence surveys indicate that the social gradient is the opposite of those for leptospirosis—that is, the much more marginalized areas were protected rather than the wealthier areas. According to Ko, this suggests that movement plays an important role in Zika transmission. At the epicenter of the Zika epidemic, he said, they carried out hospital-based surveillance for microcephaly. He reported on unpublished data that revealed at a private hospital not supported by the national health plan the prevalence of microcephaly among all newborns was 1.2 percent; at a public hospital, the rate was about 10 times higher at 12.0 percent. He suggested that much of this was driven by exposure: in the public hospital, 63.1 percent of mothers were seropositive compared to 18.8 percent of mothers from wealthier communities in the private hospital. He cautioned that, beyond these figures, the brunt of the Zika epidemic—caring for the children with neurodevelopmental problems—will be borne by the public health system.

Community-Driven Initiative for Social Equity and Urban Leptospirosis Prevention

Ko emphasized that the transmission of infectious diseases in the slums is a complex interaction of poverty, geography, and climate, but he described opportunities to identify defined structural determinants, both environmental and social, that could be targeted for intervention. Addressing open sewers and rainwater drainage are two such opportunities, he said. He noted that addressing the issue of social gradient to risk is more complex, but strategies might include a better understanding of the psychosocial factors that place young males at risk for leptospirosis, sexually transmitted infections, violence, and drug use in poor urban slum communities. He described the Fiocruz-Cornell Global Infectious Disease Training Program, a community-driven initiative for social equity and urban leptospirosis prevention that has been under way over the last 20 years in collaboration with the government of Brazil. It aims to mount multilevel interventions based on forecasting, health education to address high-risk behaviors, and targeted rodent control. This initiative reported a fourfold decrease in leptospirosis during the program. Social participation and community buy-in are keys to the success of such initiatives, he said. For example, Pau da Lima community leaders convinced the government to invest $36 million to build closed sewage systems on the periphery of the community.

TUBERCULOSIS TRANSMISSION IN CAPE TOWN, SOUTH AFRICA

Robin Wood, chief executive officer of the Desmond Tutu HIV Centre and Foundation at the University of Cape Town, focused his presentation on the transmission of TB in Cape Town, South Africa, where the country is estimated to have the highest burden of TB in the world. The city of Cape Town alone has more TB case notifications per year (around 26,000) than Canada, France, United Kingdom, and the United States combined (WHO, 2016). He said that, compared to the age-adjusted TB rates in New York City over the past 100 years (which have dropped overall, especially among young people), the same rates in Cape Town have changed very little. He reported that today there is as much TB in children and more TB among young adults in South Africa and suggested that the HIV epidemic is a contributing factor (Hermans et al., 2015).

Wood noted that, although TB was made a notifiable disease in Cape Town in 1904—a decade before it became notifiable in the United Kingdom—the massive TB burden persists despite every advance in TB control measures having been implemented in Cape Town since the beginning of the 20th century. According to cross-sectional infection rates for proportions in different age groups in Cape Town, said Wood, 20 percent of the population is infected by the time they enter school at 5 years of age, 50 percent are infected by age 14, and by adulthood, most people are either infected or have active TB disease (Wood et al., 2010).

Airborne Component of *Mycobacterium tuberculosis* Life Cycle

Wood explained that the *Mycobacterium tuberculosis* (MTB) life cycle has an airborne component. He said that the Wells-Riley equation, developed in the 1950s, can be used to predict the number of new cases of airborne infections in a steady-state, single-transmission environment (Wells, 1955). He added that the equation can be generalized to take into account multiple transmission factors and model the transmission of MTB within a given population. The modified version of the Wells-Riley equation can be used to estimate the annual risk of TB infection, he said, which is determined by the number of inhaled TB infectious quanta per year.

He highlighted three parts of the modified equation. The first part is the

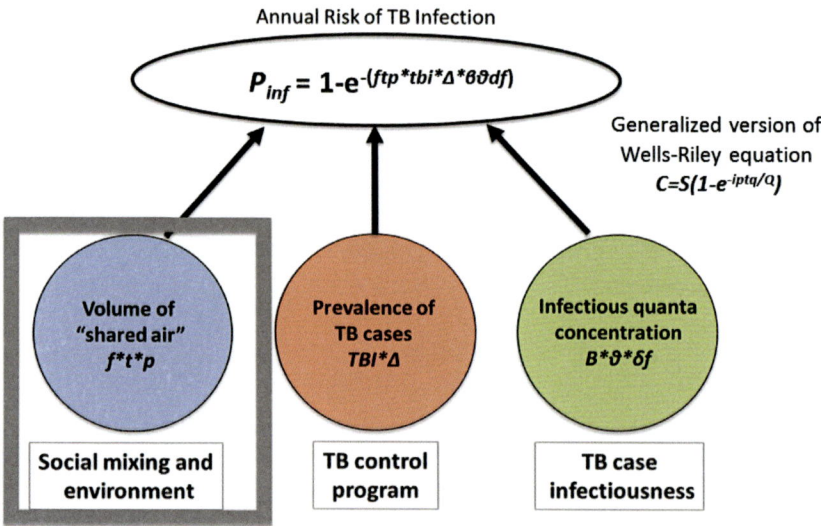

FIGURE 4-4 Modified Wells-Riley equation for estimating annual risk of tuberculosis (TB) infections using number of inhaled TB infectious quanta per year.
NOTES: The generalized Wells-Riley equation $C = S(1-e^{-iptq/Q})$ calculates number of new infected cases; i = number of infectious people; p = ventilation rate of susceptible people; q = quantum of infection; Q = constant rate of ventilation in an indoor environment; S = number of susceptible people; t = time; TB = tuberculosis.
SOURCE: Wood presentation, December 12, 2017.

volume of air breathed from others; this is relevant to an airborne disease like TB, he said, because the volume of air exchanged between people is likely a key factor that is driven by social mixing and the environment. The second part is the population prevalence of infectious TB cases, he said, which is relevant because TB control programs try to decrease prevalence by putting people onto effective therapy. The third part—the infectiousness of the range of TB cases—is also known as the infectious quanta concentration, said Wood; he noted that there is ongoing work to better understand this component of TB transmission (see Figure 4-4).

Modeling the Risk of Airborne Infectious Disease Using Exhaled Air

Wood focused more closely on the component of the modified Wells-Riley equation that represents social mixing and the environment. He described how the equation can be used to model the risk of airborne disease transmission by using measurements of exhaled air. Carbon dioxide is often used to measure ventilation, he noted, because a single person produces about 8 liters (40,000 parts per million) of carbon dioxide each minute. If the carbon dioxide level in an indoor room increases to 4,000 parts per million, he explained, then around 10 percent of every breath taken by a person in that room has been breathed out by somebody else. He added that, by using measurements of room volume, ventilation, and carbon dioxide production rate, it is possible to calculate the total amount of air that was exchanged in a room. It is also possible to calculate how long it will take for a room to reach steady-state equilibrium of carbon dioxide concentration, he said; the final steady state is defined as the carbon dioxide production of everyone in the room divided by the per-person ventilation. He noted that it takes longer to reach equilibrium in a large room and less time in a room with a greater amount of ventilation (Issarow et al., 2015).

Using Continuous Personal Carbon Dioxide Monitors to Calculate Shared Air

Wood explained that carbon dioxide disseminates rapidly, and he and his colleagues believe that carbon dioxide behaves in a similar way to the small particles (1 to 2 microns in size) that are thought to be transmitters of mycobacteria and TB. He said his team created a small device for people to wear that measures carbon dioxide levels continuously and enables location tracking, which allows researchers to calculate the amount of air exchanged between individuals in a variety of environments. He described a set of studies that used these continuous personal carbon dioxide monitors to calculate the volume of shared air in different settings and to determine if those settings reached carbon dioxide equilibrium.

Wood reported that in one study the device was used by an adolescent girl living in a relatively dense community (25,000 people in one square kilometer) as she traveled to school by taxi and public transportation and spent her day in school (Richardson et al., 2014). The researchers found that the carbon dioxide levels were dramatically different in various classrooms within the school in which she spent time. In two of those classrooms in particular, he said, the rates of rebreathed air peaked at around 0.35 to 0.375 liters per minute by the end of the classroom periods. In these two classrooms, the carbon dioxide concentrations in the rooms did not reach steady-state equilibrium during the class periods she attended, which indicates that the ventilation rates were very low. He noted that those two classrooms only had windows on one side, while the other rooms had cross flow from windows on both sides.

In another study, Wood said, the devices were used by a large group of adolescents in the township of Masiphumelele. He reported that the results showed that most of the rebreathed air was at home and in school; there was also a difference between the liters of rebreathed air in summer and winter (Wood et al., 2014). He said that in the winter, the adolescents in the study were rebreathing between 150 and 300 liters per day on average, mainly at school; in the summer, the students averaged between around 50 and 90 liters of rebreathed air per day. For reference, he estimated that most people in attendance at the workshop rebreathe around 25 liters per day.

Wood described a subsequent study that placed the carbon dioxide measurement devices throughout the township. He said that this allowed the investigators to compare concentrations of carbon dioxide with the locations of the adolescents, the locations of people who had just been diagnosed with TB, and the locations of people who had completed therapy for acute sickness of TB (Patterson et al., 2017). Wood reported that the locations of those three groups did not seem to overlap, suggesting that the people identified as *having* TB did not appear to be the same people who were *transmitting* the infection to adolescents. He said that a member of his research team created a model to integrate social contact and environmental data to evaluate TB transmission in the township (Andrews et al., 2014). He explained that, for any given age group, the model calculates the social mixing and carbon dioxide data to estimate where people are becoming infected. The results showed that between 10 and 20 percent of transmission was taking place in households, but the model estimated that among young people ages 15 to 19, more than 50 percent of transmission was taking place in schools. He attributed this to the associative nature of households—where a person meets the same people every day—versus the more generalized mixing that occurs in public spaces.

Ventilation in School Classrooms

Spurred by the finding that a high level of transmission was taking place in schools in the township of Masiphumelele, Wood said that he investigated ventilation in school classrooms. He found a study from 1924 that measured carbon dioxide levels in schools in New York City and found that they rarely exceeded 1,000 parts per million (Simpson, 1924). Wood surmised that one of the reasons the carbon dioxide concentrations were maintained at safe levels—even though the rooms appear small and crowded by modern standards—is that the classrooms had high windows with ventilation driven by temperature gradients rather than the current reliance on cross flow from windows on two sides of a room.

To illustrate the conditions of classroom ventilation in modern schools, Wood used a figure adapted from a 2008 study that plotted the correlation between mean indoor carbon dioxide concentrations against airflow rate per person in 62 naturally ventilated classrooms in Europe and North America (Santamouris et al., 2008) (see Figure 4-5). Wood noted that the

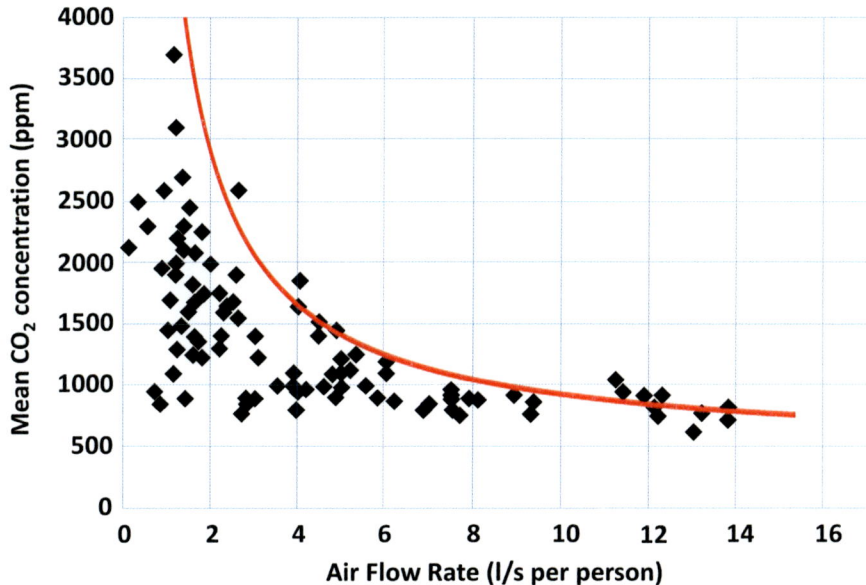

FIGURE 4-5 Correlation between the mean indoor carbon dioxide concentrations in 62 naturally ventilated classrooms and airflow per person.
NOTES: The red line represents idealized values of ventilation having reached steady-state values of carbon dioxide concentrations; x-axis is the ventilation rate per occupant; y-axis is the measured concentration of carbon dioxide (parts per million); CO_2 = carbon dioxide; l/s = liters per second; ppm = parts per million.
SOURCES: Wood presentation, December 12, 2017; Richardson et al., 2014.

idealized steady-state ventilation was rarely achieved in the classrooms surveyed in the study, as indicated by the red line he overlaid on Figure 4-5. He explained that equilibrium is achieved rapidly when airflow is high, but equilibrium is not achieved when airflow is low. He also noted that the carbon dioxide levels in the classrooms were high, reaching nearly 4,000 parts per million. Therefore, he said, people are being forced to rebreathe around 300 liters of air during an 8-hour school day. He noted that international recommendations for carbon dioxide levels in schools tend to advise a median peak carbon dioxide concentration of around 1,000 parts per million (Richardson et al., 2014).

Wood concluded by arguing that air volumes exchanged are major drivers of TB, especially in South Africa, and that rebreathing is facilitated by social mixing and environmental conditions. For example, he said that an ideal environment for TB would be an overcrowded prison where people spend 23 hours per day with no ventilation and breathe between 1,000 and 2,000 liters of other people's air per day. Wood maintained that the main role of TB control programs should be to address the prevalence of TB transmitters in the population, but he noted that it can be difficult to find the transmitters who are infecting the groups of people with the highest infection rates. Wood also suggested examining the infectiousness of TB transmitters. He explained that when social circumstances are relatively good, and people are not rebreathing large amounts of air, TB outbreaks can only be caused by superspreaders and the outbreaks do not develop into endemic disease, because the next generation will not be infectious. When there is endemic TB, he warned, the entire spectrum of MTB infectiousness can transmit disease.

DISCUSSION

Jay Siegel, recently retired chief biotechnology officer and head of scientific strategy and policy at Johnson & Johnson, noted that in Bethesda, Maryland, there is a county building code that does not require air exchange, but actually caps air exchange. He explained that when a new home is built, sealed door and air pressure tests are required to ensure that the home is airtight to minimize gas exchange to attempt to decrease energy consumption. He remarked that such construction codes have led to an increase in buildings with sick people and where carpeting or insulation are degassing volatile organic compounds. He asked Wood if such building codes are in place in South Africa or elsewhere and whether those codes are increasing the infectious disease risk.

Wood replied that in the United States there have been some extraordinary contact numbers of children in schools. To illustrate, he described a respiratory virus epidemic in Colorado where hundreds of people were infected by one person, which suggests a superspreader story, he said. He suggested that part of the problem is that architects have not been provided with the medical and disease-related reasons for not decreasing the ventilation per current trends. The building codes in South Africa, he added, require that a portion of the floor area must be open to the outdoors. He suggested that disease-related factors need to be taken into consideration and architects need to be advised about how design is important for health. Wood provided another example of the Pollsmoor Prison in Cape Town, South Africa, where hundreds of people are housed in a single room with no ventilation—that room in the prison is subject to exactly the same building code as a domestic bedroom in the same area, he said. Wood suggested that TB control programs should be tailored to social circumstances to achieve their aim of decreasing TB prevalence. If there are poor ventilation systems in places like prisons, he said, then the TB control program needs to be able to identify cases quickly to prevent rapid spread.

He elaborated that passive case-finding strategies, for example, are not suitable for groups of people with TB-HIV coinfection with rapidly progressing TB or for TB patients who are living in poor circumstances. He suggested that more active case-finding strategies should be used to look for cases that occur in those types of circumstances. He said that this was done in Cape Town in the 1970s during the lowest point of the TB epidemic, when millions of chest X-rays were carried out. He added that the TB control program was ordered to stop the campaign because it was no longer cost-effective according to global guidelines, even though it was effective for the specific context.

David Nabarro, advisor for health systems and sustainability at 4SD, suggested that the superspreader issue should be considered in every effort against infectious diseases, be it cholera, influenza, or TB. He suggested focusing on the significance of superspreaders as key individuals infected with bacteria, viruses, or other microorganisms who transmit them to an unusually large number of other people. Wood replied that superspreaders are important and disease specific; for example, he explained that in measuring the infectivity of TB individuals and measuring their production rate of appropriately sized particles, superspreaders have only been found historically because the sensitivities in systems for finding them are low. He suggested that the problem of superspreaders needs to be defined properly and disease specifically in addition to having appropriate, sensitive systems.

Wood continued that part of the success of the TB control achieved in New York was because of the spectrum of people—many people with low infectivity and a few people with high infectivity—which allowed efforts to focus on those few high-infectivity cases. In Cape Town, he explained, there is a situation of endemic TB spread in which everybody is transmitting rather than a single superspreader, because there are more than 500 TB strains in the community. Gurley noted that it is difficult to identify superspreaders for cholera, because it is related to both host infectiousness and social context.

Peter Daszak, president of EcoHealth Alliance, asked Gurley about current interventions for cholera and if new interventions will be informed by knowing more about where cases start. Gurley replied that the long-term goal of getting people safe water to drink should be pursued doggedly or progress will never be made. She noted that there is now a good vaccine for cholera, but it is not used widely enough; she explained that vaccine strategies are often based on administrative units rather than high-risk areas and populations, and that many of the current intervention strategies and systems are not flexible enough to take risk into account. If more flexibility can be cultivated, she suggested, then interventions like vaccines may help reduce hot spots of risk by addressing them at early stages and thus reducing the risk for everyone else. Nabarro asked Gurley to elaborate on the issue of water versus sanitation for cholera intervention.

Gurley replied that cholera is often spread through contaminated hands within a household, and the first person infected in a given household was probably infected by water. She said that household spread is also water related because good access to water is needed for hand washing. Sanitation is part of good infrastructure, she said, but ensuring clean water would go a long way. Nabarro responded that the delay in globally advancing sanitation is distressing and suggested that water is often put ahead of sanitation in public health. Sanitation is an integral issue in the built environment, he said, and suggested pushing for better sanitation that is not necessarily water based, such as the separation of feces, particularly children's feces and particularly during the rainy seasons.

Espinal noted that the internationally cited death toll from EVD is approximately 11,000 people, but the conclusion of one report was that the true number of people who died will never be known because the West Point slum was so complicated to deal with, and the bodies were being disposed of without being counted. He also noted that EVD was quickly contained in Nigeria, including Lagos, a huge and poor city. He asked if there are lessons to be gained regarding slums and big cities by comparing the control of EVD in Nigeria versus Liberia. Mahoney replied that there were many occult burials on an island outside of West Point. He said that the case of West Point was striking because EVD did not spread there in expected geographic ways for an infectious disease: the outbreaks were geographically tight, with a cluster around households in West Point, beyond which it did not spread much. He added that, unlike the way that cholera spreads, for example, EVD exposure was family related. Mahoney said that in the example of Nigeria they were lucky in having the right people at the right time to help mentor clinical staff, although he noted that Nigeria did experience critical issues, including a doctor strike. Mahoney said that, at one point, a contact showed up in another city, and the staff from that city called Lagos and said they had sufficient personal protective equipment and were going to see the patient. Mahoney said that they were told not to see the patient, to lock the door, and to wait for people who were experienced in managing an EVD patient; the patient was retrieved and brought back to Lagos via an 8-hour taxi ride.

He reiterated that the people managing Ebola patients need to be mentored by those with experience and said that Nigeria was fortunate to have experienced people as part of the effort. Mahoney added that Nigeria's Field Epidemiology Training Program did a great job contact tracing, that the Polio Incident Management Team was brought in to help manage the outbreak response, and that the response had a strong infrastructure of data-driven management. Mahoney outlined some lessons learned in the Nigerian response. He said that there was a program to trace EVD contact on a daily basis, but some contacts would present with the disease after several days without contact and claim that they had forgotten they were being traced; in other cases, people who were supposed to take temperatures of contacts daily were not actually doing so. From this they learned that they needed to directly observe temperature monitoring of contacts, he said.

Christopher Braden, deputy director of the National Center for Emerging and Zoonotic Infectious Diseases, CDC, asked if new technologies will enable more sensitive types of environmental sampling. Ko replied that this is a critical research need and technology is improving, but there are several barriers. He said many of the technological advances are in detection rather than processing—for example, that the volume of the infectious dose is small for toxoplasmosis and cryptosporidiosis, but processing requires 20 to 40 liters of water. Ko said that the sampling design is also challenging: exposures are highly probabilistic for highly stochastic processes, as with leptospirosis. He added that further issues are related to obtaining the sample density needed to get a signal as well as how to get the signal above the noise in a spatial grid.

Wood reported that environmental sampling is being done, but a problem is that large droplets fall out of the air and leave evidence of TB on floors and walls. However, he said that the relevance of this type of sampling to transmission is unknown, although signals can be detected. He noted that biodefense machines are used to sample large volumes of air (by cubic meter per minute) in community and health settings, and PCR has shown positive signals. He suggested that this is useful for children in classrooms, compared to other settings such as churches, because the identities of the schoolchildren in the classroom are known and they can be resampled later. Ko noted that this type of environmental pathogen sampling is somewhat locked into risk assessment, rather than linking those environmental signals and risks to human outcomes. Mahoney added that environmental sampling in work on polio has advanced far enough to track chains of transmission due to genetic clades, although he noted that this is probably unique to that virus.

Christopher Dye, director of strategy, policy, and information at the Office of the Director-General of WHO, remarked that John Snow fixed the water supply but did not recommend active surveillance; he noted that water and sanitation sectors tend to be confined to the health domain and may be reluctant to get into active surveillance. He asked if the inclusion of safe water and sanitation in the Sustainable Development Goals (SDGs) framework is an advance over the MDG framework, because the word "safe" ties health to water and sanitation in a way that was not present in the MDG era.[5] Gurley replied that John Snow may not have fixed the water supply, but he cut it off for a time while the problem was addressed. She agreed that the emphasis on safety is important and suggested that checking the veracity of sources should be incorporated going forward: that is, rather than saying "This person told me this is their water source; therefore their water is safe," better ways are needed to measure that safety. She noted that surveillance for cholera is one way to implement that, but there are many other potential ways.

Espinal concluded the discussion by remarking that the presentations underscored the importance of the International Health Regulations and the Global Health Security Agenda in ensuring that countries implement essential public health functions to contain outbreaks and emergencies. The presentations also highlighted the need for more support for research about the drivers of infectious disease, he said. He suggested there are other systemic issues at hand, noting that rainfall, climate change, and housing are related to the SDGs and that progress might be made by addressing them.

---

[5] Since the MDGs, the WHO-UNICEF Joint Monitoring Programme for Water Supply, Sanitation, and Hygiene has introduced more categories for safe water and sanitation facilities: limited, basic, or safely managed.

5

Achieving Sustainable and Health-Promoting Urban Built Environments

Session 2 of the workshop focused on effective interventions and policies aimed at achieving sustainable and health-promoting urban built environments. Prior to the session, Steve Lindsay, professor in biosciences at Durham University, England, outlined global efforts aimed at leveraging the Sustainable Development Goals (SDGs) and promoting healthy lives in urban settings. The session was moderated by Jason Corburn, director of the Institute of Urban and Regional Development and professor of city and regional planning at the University of California, Berkeley. In his presentation, Siddharth Agarwal, director of the Urban Health Resource Centre in India, explored how to build an investment case for slum upgrading and health-promoting urban environments and outlined several methods for infectious disease mitigation that have been implemented in slum environments in India. Daniele Lantagne, associate professor of civil and environmental engineering at Tufts University, discussed examples of context-specific water, sanitation, and hygiene (WASH) interventions that have been implemented successfully. Eva Harris, professor of infectious diseases and director of the Center for Global Public Health at the University of California, Berkeley, described efforts to engage communities from surveillance to policy. Her presentation focused on the Camino Verde approach to community engagement for vector control, which was the subject of a large, cluster randomized controlled trial across Nicaragua and Mexico.

GLOBAL EFFORTS TO LEVERAGE THE SUSTAINABLE DEVELOPMENT GOALS TO PROMOTE HEALTH

Steve Lindsay, professor in biosciences at Durham University, England, explored global efforts to leverage the SDGs to improve health, with a focus on health in urban built environments. He opened by describing three major infectious disease threats to urban environments: respiratory viruses, such as pandemic influenza and severe acute respiratory syndrome; *Aedes*-borne diseases, such as dengue, Zika virus disease, chikungunya, and yellow fever; and locally important diseases, such as plague and malaria in India. According to Lindsay, infectious diseases are a serious and mounting threat to the health of people living in towns and cities around the world, and he suggested that this threat remains underappreciated on an international level. He said that the *Aedes aegypti* mosquito is an urban vector of chief concern. He noted that dengue fever, for example, is a predominantly urban disease that is increasing worldwide, with an estimated increase in age-standardized dengue cases of nearly 450 percent between 1990 and 2013 (Vos et al., 2015). Lindsay predicted that the number of dengue cases will continue to increase, given the predicted increase in the distribution of *Aedes aegypti* in large human populations around the world. He warned: "We are so ignorant about the true distribution of this mosquito, this fantastic vector of arboviruses." Lindsay also expressed serious concern about the ability to control a disease such as yellow fever if it moves into one of the megacities in South America.

Global Initiatives to Mitigate the Risk of Infectious Diseases in Urban Environments

After outlining some of the major infectious disease threats to urban built environments, Lindsay turned to global initiatives aimed at mitigating the risk of such diseases. He said that the SDGs provide an opportunity for improving control of infectious diseases in urban settings because they provide a reason for action. He suggested that, because the SDGs govern and support international documents, they have the potential to contribute to more focused policy documents, to the reorienting of organization of policies going forward, and ultimately to a cultural shift toward multidisciplinary solutions to complex problems.

Lindsay focused on six of the SDGs that he considers potentially helpful in improving the control of infectious diseases:

- SDG 1: No poverty
- SDG 3: Good health and well-being
- SDG 6: Clean water and sanitation

- SDG 11: Sustainable cities and communities
- SDG 13: Climate action
- SDG 17: Partnerships for the goals

He said that the SDGs were influential in helping to develop the new global vector control response from the World Health Organization (WHO). He explained that WHO had a previous global strategy for dealing with vector-borne diseases—a multidisciplinary approach called the Global Strategic Framework for Integrated Vector Management (WHO, 2004)—but the global Zika pandemic, coupled with the SDGs, caused WHO to reexamine global vector control and to produce its Global Vector Control Response 2017–2030, which provides a new strategy to strengthen vector control worldwide through increased capacity, improved surveillance, better coordination, and integrated action across sectors and diseases (WHO, 2017a).

According to Lindsay, another illustration of how the SDGs have helped to develop global health policy is related to SDG 11 (sustainable cities and communities). He said that SDG 11 catalyzed the United Nations Human Settlements Programme's (UN-Habitat's) New Urban Agenda, which supports towns and cities in developing strategies to become more resilient to the threats of natural hazards (UN-Habitat, 2016b). Although the new agenda mentions health and vector-borne diseases, he said, much of the current thinking within this field is focused on hazard threats, such as rising sea levels and earthquakes, rather than the threat of infectious diseases. Lindsay highlighted the enormous potential for the health sector to link productively with the group of people who developed the New Urban Agenda. Lindsay also noted that other initiatives flow from the new agenda, including the Global Alliance for Urban Crises[1] and The Rockefeller Foundation's 100 Resilient Cities.[2] He suggested that those initiatives could also provide opportunities for people working in health to link with people working on promoting resilience to physical, social, and economic challenges in specific cities. He suggested focusing on engaging the mayors of cities and towns, because they have power, access to financing, and the facilities to take action. He emphasized that infections such as *Aedes*-borne diseases are environmental illnesses and contended that health should be integrated with work that is already under way to develop these new ideas and initiatives, rather than being a separate strand.

---

[1] The Global Alliance for Urban Crises is available at www.urbancrises.org (accessed February 10, 2018).
[2] The Rockefeller Foundation's 100 Resilient Cities is available at www.smartresilient.com/100-resilient-cities-rockefeller-foundation (accessed February 10, 2018).

Translating Global Initiatives into Local Action: A Focus on Vector Control

Lindsay discussed some ongoing efforts to translate global initiatives into local action. He explained that WHO's Global Vector Control Response 2017–2030 can be envisioned as a temple requiring four key pillars to attain locally adapted and sustainable vector control (see Figure 5-1). Two of its four pillars are to strengthen intersectoral and intrasectoral action and collaboration and to engage and mobilize communities. He said that addressing those two pillars is a challenge because the function of intersectoral committees is contingent on commitment at the highest national or

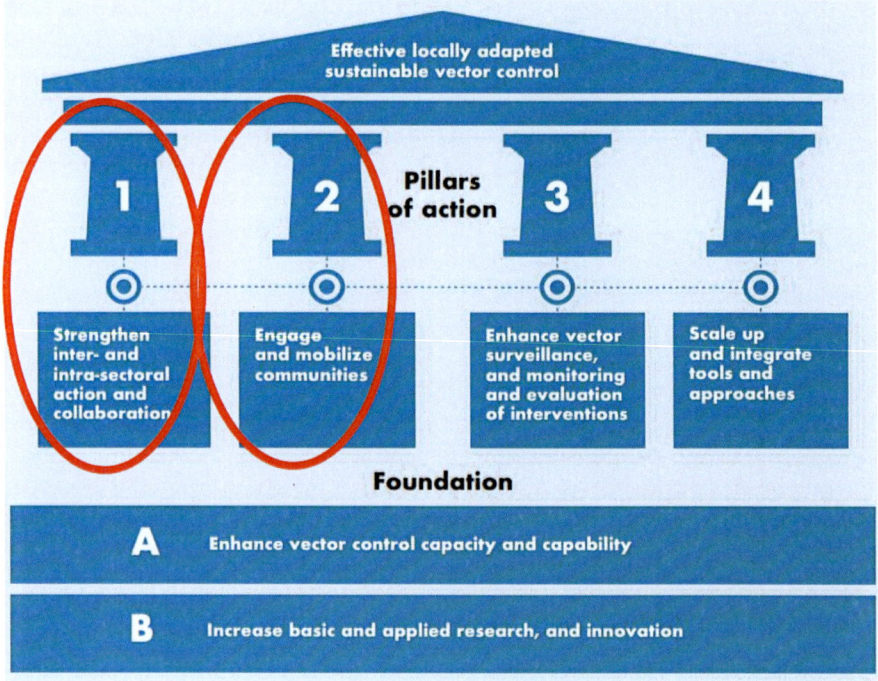

FIGURE 5-1 Response framework in the World Health Organization's (WHO's) Global Vector Control Response 2017–2030 to reduce the burden and threat of vector-borne diseases affecting humans.
SOURCES: Lindsay presentation, December 13, 2017; adapted from WHO, 2017a. Reprinted from *Global Vector Control Response 2017—2030*, page ix, Copyright (2017).

local level. He maintained that this is the key for turning policy into action. He said that a national steering committee for improving control of vector-borne diseases, for example, must collaborate with agencies outside of the government ministries of agriculture, finance, environment, and others, as well as collaborate with the private sector, with community groups, and with nongovernmental organizations.

Lindsay said there is a set of tried and tested technologies for control of vector-borne diseases, including insecticide-treated bed nets, fogging, indoor residual spraying, and larval source management. He also noted other underexplored opportunities that are founded on better appreciating the importance of environmental management and city design. For example, he said, the immature stages of *Aedes aegypti* are carried in water storage containers, used tires, solid waste, and elsewhere. To eliminate aquatic habitats for the vector and reduce the number of adult mosquitos, he explained, strategies that may discourage people from storing water include removing tires, improving waste management, and providing reliable piped water. These types of strategies will not solve the problem, he conceded, but he suggested that they can contribute to the overall control of *Aedes*-borne diseases in the future, as well as improving people's living conditions in the present.

Making intersectoral collaboration sustainable is one of the biggest challenges of the century, according to Lindsay, but he suggested that effectively controlling infectious disease in urban environments will need to include collaborating and gleaning lessons learned from organizations outside the health sector. He further suggested that turning policy into action will require "breaking the mold" within the health sector by engaging with communities and with nonhealth sectors. The ethos should be health in all policies, he said, not just the deployment of tools (WHO, 2013). Lindsay cautioned that establishing intersectoral collaboration may be challenging against the current background of weak health systems and the unknown effectiveness of existing interventions, particularly for interventions against *Aedes*-borne diseases. He also mentioned the lack of research and investment into methods for controlling, intervening, and monitoring and evaluation of these diseases. In cities in tropical and subtropical regions, he suggested that efforts should focus on controlling *Aedes*-borne diseases. Lindsay commended the Sudan National Intersectoral Committee for Vector Control as an instructive example of a successful and effective interdisciplinary approach to controlling malaria by removing aquatic breeding habitats in Khartoum, Sudan. He concluded by reiterating that there is a "golden" opportunity to collaborate outside the health sector by working with the people driving the New Urban Agenda, who are actively engaged in helping city planners design the cities for the future all over the world.

During the discussion that followed Lindsay's presentation, Jonna

Mazet, executive director of the One Health Institute at the University of California, Davis, asked Lindsay to elaborate on the success in Sudan and how the different sectors were brought together. She noted that tangible success stories are relatively rare in the One Health space, which involves collaboration among human, animal, and environmental health sectors. Lindsay explained that the Sudan National Intersectoral Committee for Vector Control had full political support, some financing, and an effective and dynamic person in charge and running the committee. He explained that they searched for and eliminated the location of the aquatic habitats; for example, they replaced leaking pipes that were relics of poor and aged British engineering. When they found that builders were not destroying the water supplies used for making cement on construction sites after the work was complete, said Lindsay, they took advantage of a bylaw outlawing this practice and went around the city destroying the water supply habitat. Similarly, he said that they required agricultural fields around the city to be free of water for a certain number of days each week. He added that they originally started to fine farmers who did not comply, which outraged the farmers, but when they explained the rationale for this decision, the farmers agreed to cooperate. Lindsay also said that they had a "malaria day" for schools in Khartoum, and schoolchildren were asked to find and eliminate a small aquatic habitat of some kind. Regardless of the sustainability or effectiveness of that intervention, he said, it was a worthwhile way to engage and communicate with the community.

Lindsay noted that his vision may be broader than the One Health concept—at least as it is construed in the United Kingdom, where it generally refers to veterinary diseases or infections coming from domestic livestock to humans. He said that he is interested in further understanding the infectious disease dynamics in populations of wild animals—not only domesticated animals—to better understand spillover events into humans. Mazet added that the implementation of large-scale One Health projects is sometimes impeded by the practical human nature problems and balancing concerns among different ministries.

David Nabarro, advisor for health and sustainability at 4SD, remarked that the multisectoral, interdisciplinary approach espoused by Lindsay is the same approach envisaged when the SDG agenda was first produced: a universal approach that applies anywhere in the world, involves interconnected thinking and action, includes all sectors of society during implementation, and involves partnering as well as integrated action. He suggested conceptualizing how to advance this approach. For example, he suggested that the work on *Aedes*-borne arboviruses and other vector-borne diseases could be linked to other activities—such as child nutrition or access to water and sanitation—without necessarily losing or weakening the emphasis on those particular arboviral diseases. Nabarro predicted that this approach, in line with the SDGs, will be available in many more urban settings. He cautioned that overemphasizing vector-borne disease projects may constrain thinking. Instead, he suggested encouraging interdisciplinary and multi-stakeholder movements for health and seeking ways to integrate work on specific problems, like the arboviruses, to initiatives that are perhaps larger or differently shaped. Lindsay replied that his concern is overloading the system by making it impossible for committees to function and creating an unwieldy system by trying to do everything. He clarified that he is not trying to oversell *Aedes*-borne diseases, but to encourage people to reflect about what can be done in urban centers to reduce that risk as well as addressing other locally determined priorities.

BUILDING AN INVESTMENT CASE FOR HEALTH-PROMOTING URBAN ENVIRONMENTS

To explore strategies for building an investment case for upgrading slums and promoting health in urban environments, Siddharth Agarwal drew upon his work as director of the Urban Health Resource Centre in India. He said there is a large, disadvantaged, and increasingly urban population in India that contributes inexpensive labor to the growing economy of India. This population includes women and children, he noted, with child-bearing migrant girls facing particular risks. Agarwal explained that this group faces a host of difficulties in accessing education, social opportunities, and other services in slum environments and, in many cases, they have little awareness of the opportunities and services that are available to them. These disadvantages are compounded by restrictions on their freedom of movement and weak social networks, he added.

Agarwal maintained that it is critical to improve infection prevention in the slum environments where these types of disadvantaged populations reside and where pathogens thrive. He suggested that investing in the health and well-being of these slum populations benefits the urban area at large and contributes to national-level economic growth, because the urban component of the gross domestic product of many developing countries is growing faster than the rural component. By neglecting to address infectious disease transmission in slums, he noted that pathogens will continue to thrive, which will contribute to increased health care expenditures and a less productive workforce. Agarwal said that it can be difficult to finance investment in slums, either in the form of action research or time-bound funding, because there are so many unknowns and funders are often risk averse. However, he emphasized that these populations are living their lives at risk and argued that that they deserve a courageous approach to investment aimed at improving their lives.

> **BOX 5-1**
> **Examples of Methods to Mitigate Infectious Diseases in Slum Environments in India**
>
> - Qualitative assessment of urban health inequities by women's groups
> - Spatial mapping of all slums
> - Disaggregating urban data to expose inequities
> - Gentle demand-side negotiation with authorities
> - Establishment of a revolving community fund for health and social needs
> - Enhanced access to voter identification
> - Empowerment through women's groups
> - Encouraging women's livelihoods
> - Empowerment through youth groups
>
> SOURCE: Agarwal presentation, December 13, 2017.

Methods for Mitigating Infectious Diseases in Slums

Agarwal outlined a set of methods that have been implemented in India to mitigate infectious diseases in slum environments (see Box 5-1). He explained three methods to specifically help identify and assess slum conditions and inequities that would incite action. In the first method described by Agarwal, representatives from local women's groups are engaged to assess living conditions across several slums using a qualitative adaptation of WHO's Urban Health Equity Assessment and Response Tool (Urban HEART).[3] With this tool, the women use color-coded dots to denote their assessment of each indicator. He said that this method drives action in slums, for example, by encouraging households to build low-cost latrines or encouraging hand washing with soap and water. Agarwal further described the method of spatial mapping of all of the listed and unlisted slums in a city. He highlighted the significance of identifying and mapping unlisted slums because, according to government estimates, around 50 percent of slums in India are unlisted (NSSO, 2010). He added that mapping of at-risk populations, including seasonal and recent migrant clusters, is an integral strategy of India's National Urban Health Mission. Another method discussed by Agarwal is disaggregating data at the national and state levels to provide more insight into existing inequities and disparities in indicators,

---

[3] WHO's Urban HEART is available at www.who.int/kobe_centre/measuring/urbanheart/en (accessed February 10, 2018).

such as under-5-years-of-age mortality and living space density (which contributes to the transmission of infectious disease).

Agarwal also explained methods for communities to be active and take ownership in this issue. He described that gentle negotiation through community requests helps community groups to petition their local authorities and municipal corporations to improve the environmental conditions in slums by building water supply or sewage systems, for example. The groups are encouraged to maintain a paper trail and persevere with tact in their negotiations to receive the government resources for their communities, he said. Another method, said Agarwal, is to establish revolving community funds for health exigencies. Community groups manage their own revolving funds, he said, and they are trained to maintain records of loans provided for needs such as education, toilet construction, or starting a small business. He also added that the method to increase access to voter identification and proof of address for disadvantaged populations imbues people with greater power to express themselves to political leaders.

The final set of methods focuses on empowerment of vulnerable populations in India. Agarwal highlighted the approach of empowering women and girls in a largely male-dominated society. He suggested that empowering women by providing them with social support enhances their ability to care for themselves and their families, which in turn contributes to infection prevention in their homes and communities. Agarwal explained another method of encouraging women's livelihoods, which focuses on providing women with vocational training, such as tailoring and stitching, selling vegetables in markets, or establishing slum convenience stores. This strategy provides women with additional resources to help care for the health and well-being of themselves and their families, he said. Finally, Agarwal highlighted the importance of empowering young people to enhance their self-esteem, improve their lives, and contribute actively to their communities. He suggested that investing in the next generation is especially relevant in countries like India, where the population of young people is enormous.

Agarwal reported that India now has an urban health policy in place, but its ongoing implementation has been slow. He noted that the policy encourages intersectoral coordination at both the municipal and community levels to promote overall well-being and health and to reduce the risk of infectious disease. He said that in some slums and informal settlements there have already been glimpses of improvement in access to services such as toilets, sewage lines, electricity supplies, water supplies, garbage removal, and paved streets. He described the specific example of a successful 5-year campaign by community women's groups and youth groups that convinced civic authorities to build a permanent bridge over a large drain at the entrance to a slum, which directly improved the lives of 120,000 residents. Agarwal urged the group to take action toward infectious disease prevention by focusing on building the capabilities and self-reliance of slum residents and providing them with a voice to change their circumstances.

FIT-FOR-CONTEXT WATER, SANITATION, AND HYGIENE INTERVENTIONS

In her presentation on fit-for-context WASH interventions, Daniele Lantagne, associate professor of civil and environmental engineering at Tufts University, opened by suggesting that the narrative around WASH needs to be changed. She explained that there tend to be two primary WASH narratives. The first is an urban high-income water narrative, she said, where there is piped, treated infrastructure that delivers water directly to people's taps 24 hours per day, 7 days per week, and in which children are healthy and happy. The second is a primarily rural, low-income water narrative, she continued, in which people collect water from an unimproved open source and store it in a questionable storage container in the home. Within this second narrative, she said, there is a tendency to assume that providing WASH infrastructure is not yet feasible. This narrative focuses on strategies such as providing improved water sources, working with people to treat their water at the household level with chlorine or filters, providing a latrine to separate waste from the environment, and promoting hand washing. Lantagne suggested that slums do not fit neatly into either of those two narratives; she called for moving beyond those narratives to nuance and specificity for context.

Lantagne provided some historical context for WASH interventions. She explained that three types of organisms cause diarrhea at a general level: bacteria, such as those that cause cholera and typhoid; protozoa, such as *Cryptosporidium* and *Giardia lamblia*; and viruses, such as rotavirus and norovirus. She said that bacteria can be inactivated by chlorine and other disinfectants and that chlorine and other disinfectants can remove the bacteria and most viruses from water, but protozoan oocysts are chlorine resistant. She added that filtration can remove bacteria and larger protozoa from water, but filtration cannot remove viruses because they are too small. Treating water to remove all three of these organism types generally involves combined treatment of filtration plus chlorination, Lantagne said. She explained that combined treatment was the strategy used to successfully reduce infectious disease transmission across the United States and Europe during the "sanitation revolution" (approximately between 1890 and 1930). In Philadelphia, for example, she said that the number of typhoid cases peaked at around 10,000 in 1906, at which point drinking water filtration began and drove a log reduction[4] in the number of cases to around 1,000 within about 5 years. When chlorination of drinking water was introduced in the city in 1913, she added, it drove a further reduction in cases to just over 100 by 1930 (Matossian, 1997).

Urbanization, Slums, and WASH Infrastructure

Lantagne explained that the prevailing narrative was to replicate the type of combined WASH strategy used in Philadelphia by building infrastructure within developing, low-income countries. She said that infrastructure does create huge advantages, such as the widespread provision of reliable quality water, which leads to disease reduction and improved hygiene. However, she maintained that infrastructure is not appropriate for all contexts, because it requires political stability and large amounts of public funding. To illustrate, she said that the Deer Island wastewater treatment plant in Boston, Massachusetts, cost $4 billion to build and has operating costs of $300 million per year—the cost of sewage treatment in Boston is double the cost of its water, she added. She explained that infrastructure also needs land tenure that is located in conducive terrain, as well as population density and stability of population numbers—populations cannot be increasing or decreasing too quickly, she said.

Many slums cannot meet the prerequisite conditions for WASH infrastructure, Lantagne said. She explained that urbanization is driving increases in populations that are happening so quickly that it is difficult to install hard infrastructure to accommodate the rate of growth. For example, London urbanized from 1 million people to 6 to 7 million (roughly where it remains today) over a period of around 50 years between 1830 and 1890, which allowed time for infrastructure to catch up to the growth (Bairoch and Goertz, 1986). In contrast, Asia and Africa are rapidly urbanizing in the space of 20 years, with cities like Shanghai growing by at least 10 million people (UN DESA, 2015).

Lantagne noted that China is managing its urban growth through a top-down centralized scientific approach that includes rolling out identical water and wastewater treatment plants on a daily basis. However, in areas such as sub-Saharan Africa, some countries were unable to meet the Millennium Development Goal target of reducing by half the number of people without access to safe water and sanitation. In many of those countries, she said, three-quarters or more of their urban populations are living in slums with unknown land tenure (see Figure 5-2). She noted that the type of strategy used in China to roll out water and wastewater treatment

---

[4] Each log reduction indicates a 10-fold reduction in colony-forming units of microbes; a 2-log reduction would further reduce colony-forming units by 100, and so forth.

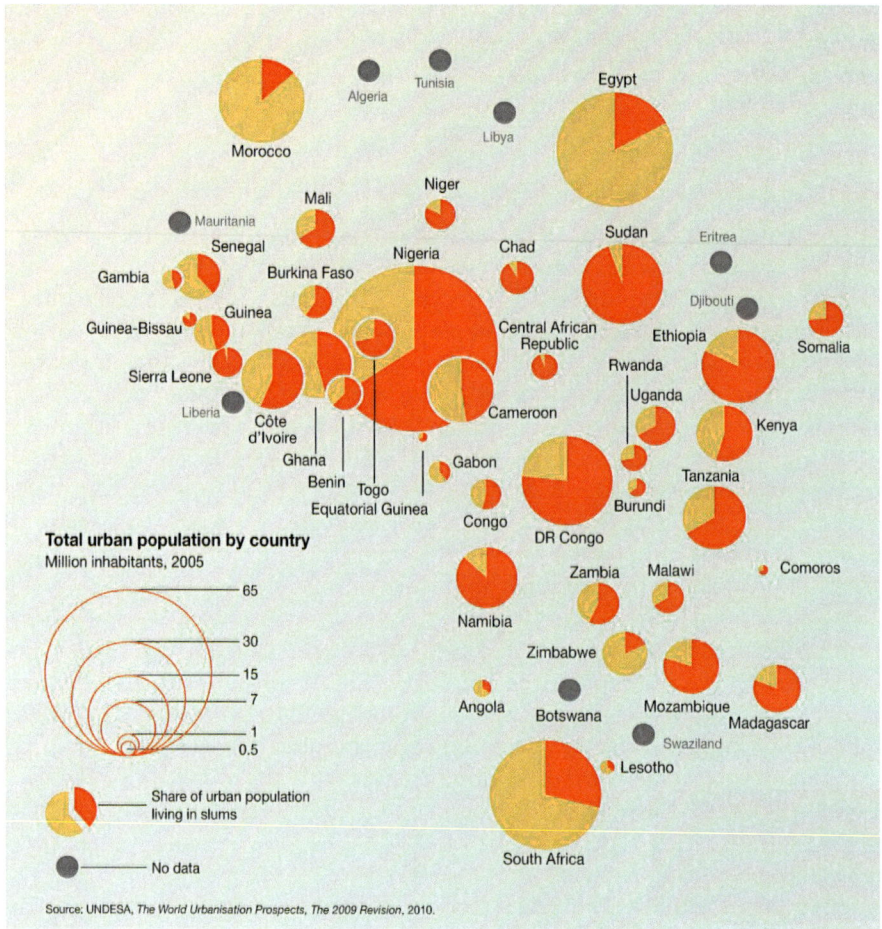

FIGURE 5-2 The proportion of urban populations living in slums in African countries.
NOTE: UN-HABITAT defines a slum household as a group of individuals living under the same roof in an urban area who lack one or more of the following: 1. Durable housing of a permanent nature that protects against extreme climate conditions. 2. Sufficient living spaces, which means not more than three people sharing the same room. 3. Easy access to safe water in sufficient amounts at an affordable price. 4 Access to adequate sanitation in the form of a private or public toilet shared by a reasonable number of people. 5. Security of tenure that prevents forced evictions.
SOURCES: Lantagne presentation, December 13, 2017; Pravettoni, UNEP/GRID-Arendal, 2011.

for rapidly growing populations is not yet feasible in many such places. She underscored the need to find ways to address slum populations in the interim until it is possible to build in reliable infrastructure.

Water, Sanitation, and Hygiene Interventions in Slums

Lantagne provided some specific examples of WASH programming and interventions in slums that have been successful in addressing water supply, water treatment, and the sanitation chain. She also described an example of a WASH intervention carried out in an emergency response context.

Water Supply Interventions

Lantagne said that water kiosks have been a success in improving water supply. She explained that the kiosk operators, who are typically in the commercial sector and not externally funded, usually obtain centrally treated water that is trucked in and stored in large containers. Water is typically sold to customers in 3-gallon containers, she said, and reported that these types of kiosks are now opening up in Haiti, Indonesia, and across Africa. She described a study in Port-au-Prince, Haiti, which found 1,300 kiosks in the city, over half of which had opened in the previous year, and most of which were obtaining water to sell from a franchise of four large providers (Patrick et al., 2017). She reported that 91 percent of the kiosks were selling water that met WHO standards for *Escherichia coli*. However, she noted that the expansion of kiosks gives rise to questions about the role of recontamination of water in households, about preserving water safety throughout the storage chain, and about the role of external funding. For example, she said, there are questions about how external funding should be used to leverage increases in water safety and whether increases in government regulations should be put in place to ensure safety throughout the water chain.

Water Treatment Interventions

Lantagne also described several successful water treatment interventions. In an ideal situation, she said, water is treated centrally, and the population receives water that can be used without further treatment. But when this is not possible, she added, water can be treated at the point of collection or at the point of use. She explained that as treatment becomes more centralized—that is, as it moves from point-of-use to point-of-collection to centralized water treatment—the amount of behavior change asked of the population decreases. More behavior change is asked of people who must treat their own water at the household (point-of-use) or community (point-of-collection) level, she added.

According to Lantagne, the distribution of locally branded safe storage containers is an example of point-of-use water treatment that has been successful in urban and rural areas of Haiti that were affected by the earthquake and cholera. Each container has a tap and a liquid chlorine solution, she said, and they are distributed by community health workers. At the height of the cholera epidemic in 2010, around three-quarters of households (15,000 households) were reached with this program, but by 2014, the number of households reached had decreased to around one half (Wilner et al., 2017). Although this decline indicates a decrease in sustainability, she said, the program's overall reach demonstrates that success is possible through community outreach and the use of appropriate products. However, she noted that it can be difficult to scale up such a program without large numbers of trained community health workers.

Lantagne described a program called Dispensers as an example of a point-of-collection intervention, as well as an illustration of how the same intervention can have different results depending on implementation quality in different settings. She explained that the program aims to reduce the need for behavior change by providing a tank of chlorine next to a community source of water, so that people can treat their water when they collect it. She reported that the program was evaluated in different emergency contexts in Haiti, Senegal, and Sierra Leone, with results highlighting the importance of context and implementation. Two countries (Sierra Leone and Haiti) had almost no use of the program, while Senegal had almost 100 percent use (Yates et al., 2015). She suggested that this disparity was caused by a set of implementation factors, such as having experienced staff, having appropriate training, having materials in the right language, and ensuring that the dispenser's engineering was functional. She cautioned that there are no silver-bullet interventions in WASH, only interventions that are appropriate for a specific context and that must be implemented well to be successful.

Sanitation Chain Interventions

To discuss successful sanitation chain interventions, Lantagne explained that people with access to modern sewage systems have the benefit of not having to deal with their own waste—it is flushed down a toilet and passes through a treatment plant and is shipped away. Within such a system, she said, large amounts of wasted clean water and large amounts of nutrients from urine and feces are not repurposed for agricultural use. In places without a modern sewage system, she explained, people rely on a sanitation chain of collection, treatment, and reuse.

Lantagne described the Fresh Life program in Kibera of Nairobi, Kenya, which provides central facilities for people to defecate.[5] The waste is collected in buckets and trucked to a waste facility treatment plant, she said, where recovered nutrients from the waste are eventually used in agriculture and, to a lesser extent, the waste is used to generate electricity. She added that Sanivation, another program in Kenya, uses a model of customer-oriented waste collection. People who join the program receive a type of home toilet and have their waste collected from the home regularly, she said, and the waste is treated using ultraviolet light and heat to transform it into briquettes sold as affordable fuel for cooking.

Emergency Response Interventions

Lantagne described emergency response work carried out with a WASH cluster in Syria, where more than 95 percent of the population had access to pipe-treated safe drinking water and sanitation in 2009. The conflict caused a rapid decline in access to the network water source, she reported, from 22 percent in 2016 to 15 percent in 2017 (Sikder et al., 2018). She noted that access varies by subdistrict, and in some areas the infrastructure is being deliberately targeted for destruction. She explained that Syria also has a private trucked water network that sells water. The majority of the population is now dependent on trucked water, she said, and the proportion of the population dependent on trucked water has increased from 77 percent of the population in 2016 to 83 percent of the population in 2017 (Sikder et al., 2018). In an effort to improve the safety of trucked water, she said, a United Nations Children's Fund intervention is providing chlorine to treat the water that is being delivered. According to Lantagne, a barrier the intervention has faced is getting the chlorine across the border into the country.

Suggested Ways Forward

Lantagne closed by recapitulating her call for a paradigm shift in the WASH narrative. She suggested moving beyond the existing WASH narratives to reach people in slums and focusing on the provision of decentralized WASH services in areas without hard infrastructure. These efforts could be strengthened, she said, by providing the necessary training and education to the people implementing the programs, as well as to the program recipients. She also suggested supporting private-sector initiatives—particularly within water interventions—to be able to achieve sufficient scale. Moving forward, there are short-term questions about decision making for interventions, she said, and longer-term questions about how to ensure programs'

---

[5] Sanergy manages Fresh Life programs in several informal settlements in Nairobi, Kenya.

sustainability over time and how to establish hard infrastructure where it is lacking. She suggested a dual focus on both the short- and long-term issues.

ENGAGING COMMUNITIES: FROM SURVEILLANCE TO POLICY

Eva Harris, professor of infectious diseases and director of the Center for Global Public Health at the University of California, Berkeley, offered her vision of the concept of engaging communities in addressing *Aedes*-borne arboviral diseases, such as dengue and Zika. Her presentation focused on an experience with community engagement in a pilot program that led to a large-scale trial, but she began by discussing the particular threat posed by *Aedes*-borne diseases. She reported that mosquitos kill an estimated 725,000 people each year worldwide, killing more people than other humans (475,000), snakes (50,000), and rabid dogs (25,000) (Gates, 2014). The *Aedes aegypti* mosquito is distributed widely across the globe, she noted (Kraemer et al., 2015) (see Figure 5-3). The *Aedes* mosquito population grows and their larvae develop in clean water around people's homes, she explained, and its proliferation is compounded by the behavioral ecology of 21st-century urbanization in tropical cities, especially issues of water and garbage management. Although there are a few notable examples of successful vector control to prevent *Aedes*-transmitted diseases, they have been difficult to sustain (Achee et al., 2015; Morrison et al., 2008; Wilder-Smith et al., 2017), and many programs have focused primarily on chemical control, which to Harris, have been problematic because of possible unintended health effects. As efforts in vector control have been insufficient, dengue, Zika, and chikungunya viruses continue to spread worldwide.

Changing Attitudes Toward Community Involvement in Interventions

To strengthen vector control efforts, Harris has been exploring ways to include communities in controlling the *Aedes* vector. Harris said that there has historically been somewhat of a bias against community involvement interventions; she suggested that this may be from a lack of data about their effectiveness, as it can be difficult to measure and quantify the effect of such programs. For example, she reported that a 2007 review found only weak evidence that community-based dengue control programs alone and in combination with other control activities can enhance the effectiveness of dengue control programs (Heintze et al., 2007). However, she noted a shift toward recognizing that communities can be involved in a productive way. She cited a meta-review which concluded that the best practice when designing interventions is to use a community-based integrated approach

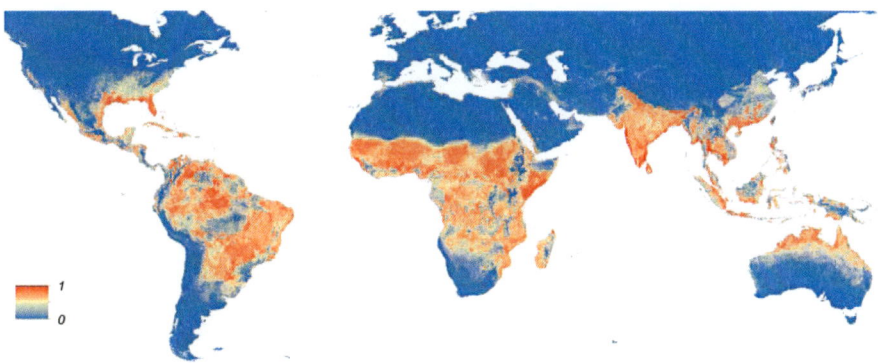

FIGURE 5-3 Global map of the predicted distribution of the *Aedes aegypti* mosquito.
NOTE: The map depicts the probability of occurrence (from 0 blue to 1 red) at a spatial resolution of 5 km × 5 km.
SOURCES: Harris presentation, December 13, 2017; Kraemer et al., 2015.

tailored to local epidemiology and sociocultural settings and combined with educational programs (Erlanger et al., 2008).

The paucity of research on this topic gives rise to questions about how to engage and motivate communities effectively, said Harris. To explore this, she described a couple of initiatives that have been implemented over the past decade that are variations on the theme of community-based participatory research. She explained that the Special Program for Research and Training in Tropical Diseases carried out an eco-bio-social initiative between 2006 and 2011 to support work on the control of vector-borne dengue in Asia and Chagas disease in Latin America (Gürtler and Yadon, 2015; Sommerfeld and Kroeger, 2012). She reported that the initiative led to new country-specified approaches and research outputs. The Pan American Health Organization's EGI-Dengue concept[6] promotes an integrated approach that includes a social communication component, she added. In Cuba, she reported that researchers used a structured format to investigate a more vertical approach to community involvement in dengue vector control using randomized controlled trials, which they found effective in embedding community empowerment strategies into routine vector control programs (Castro et al., 2012; Vanlerberghe et al., 2009).

---

[6] Commonly referred to by its Spanish acronym EGI-Dengue (*Estrategia de gestión integrada*) but is also known as the Integrated Management Strategy for Prevention and Control of Dengue. It is available at iris.paho.org/xmlui/handle/123456789/34860 (accessed March 8, 2018).

Applying the Camino Verde Approach for Sustainable Control of the *Aedes* Vector

Harris said that efforts are now oriented toward taking community engagement concepts that have been defined over the past 10 to 15 years and combining them with technology tools to allow real-time data to be captured. This allows for communities to autonomously measure and be motivated by their own progress, she said, as well as making the information collected available for reports and for country-level analysis. To illustrate such an approach, she described the Camino Verde ("Green Path") initiative, which was designed to prevent dengue and to examine community mobilization for sustainable control of the *Aedes* vector.

Camino Verde uses an epidemiological framework and methodology that had been applied in 50 different countries over 30 years to measure and to bring community data into policy, explained Harris.[7] It also incorporates the care group model approach, she said, in which facilitators work with community volunteers, who in turn work directly with individual households and residents (Perry et al., 2015). In Camino Verde, she said, the care group model was adapted into a strategy called socializing evidence for participatory action (SEPA), which was then applied to the dengue problem in Nicaragua.

Socializing Evidence for Participatory Action

Harris explained that in Camino Verde's SEPA strategy, small community teams formed groups called health brigades (*Brigadas SEPA*) and received training in pesticide-free vector control. Community leaders (*brigadistas*) then visit households to educate people about the threat of dengue and the life cycle of the *Aedes* mosquito, she said. Harris argued that the best way to engage and motivate communities is with their own data and evidence. She said that, rather than giving instructions, it is better to help communities identify their own evidence for a problem—for example, larva in water near the home—and figure out how to solve it. She maintained that this is more effective because community members are more engaged with the knowledge and with their own solutions to their own problems.

Harris explained that the SEPA strategy has three levels of intervention to help engage and motivate communities: house interventions, within-neighborhood (barrio) interventions, and interbarrio interventions. She noted that public health interventions often instruct people to get rid of mosquitos in and around their homes by eliminating standing water, clean-

---

[7] Details about Camino Verde are available at caminoverde.ciet.org/en/sepa (accessed February 10, 2018).

ing storage barrels, and applying other methods, but she suggested that this does not provide people with real motivation to carry out those onerous tasks. As part of Camino Verde, reported Harris, they held discussions with community members who told them that they wanted the underlying knowledge to understand why those kinds of actions are needed. To address this request, said Harris, the program began a campaign to educate people about the mosquito life cycle (from eggs to larvae to pupae to mosquito in about 8 to 10 days). She said they explained to the community that taking action to eliminate breeding sites just once every 8 days can cut the mosquito life cycle without using pesticides or chemicals. This type of explanation made sense to people, said Harris. Because they understood the rationale, she added, they were no longer offended that they were being asked to get rid of the old tires they owned. This in turn generated community-led solutions, she noted, such as filling these old tires with dirt to create stairways, bridges, or planters. Harris also described some of the program's barrio-level interventions, such as reducing key breeding sites in public areas, hosting barrio fairs and cleanup campaigns, and engaging schoolchildren in educational activities and games.

Camino Verde Pilot Phase

Harris reported that during Camino Verde's pilot phase they carried out an observational study in Nicaragua through a tripartite cycle of evidence gathering, analysis/planning, and intervention that was repeated and refined over 4 years (2004 to 2008). She said that evidence was obtained through entomology to gather knowledge of mosquito breeding receptacles, through surveys of knowledge and behavior, and through serology to measure antidengue antibodies in children's saliva. She explained that the latter is a noninvasive epidemiological approach to quantify infection rates; measuring infection is useful, she said, because people with asymptomatic infection are at higher risk of developing more severe disease when infected for a second time.[8] During the analysis and planning component, she said the data were analyzed and the evidence was relayed back to the community during discussions. Communities were heavily involved in the intervention component, she added, by using the evidence they were provided to create their own mosquito control strategies, communication strategies, and neighborhood brigade activities.

Harris reported that the lessons learned from the pilot phase formed the basis of a large cluster randomized controlled trial in two countries that quantified the effectiveness of community mobilization for dengue

---

[8] Paired samples gathered before and after the epidemic were used to examine the increase in antibody titers.

prevention as part of its methodology (Andersson et al., 2015). According to Harris, the following key lessons were identified:

- Evidence is critical for dialogue and reflection with residents that risk exists in their own homes, that they can control the vector in their own environment, and that integrated neighborhood action is needed.
- Socialization and dialogue about the evidence at the household and neighborhood levels can generate interventions from a cost–benefit perspective.
- Beyond motivation, the SEPA process aims for households and communities to responsibly assume control of their own health—prevention is an empowering approach.
- External actions are generated from the knowledge and experience of the communities themselves; there are no fixed, one-size-fits-all solutions; the practice is specific to each neighborhood.
- Every community is a vast microcosm, but there are certain common principles. Rather than issue instructions, provide communities with evidence and concepts they can translate into action in a way that makes sense for their own community.
- Community responsibility materializes organically; effectiveness and sustainability depend on local management and autonomy of SEPA brigades.

Camino Verde Cluster Randomized Controlled Trials

Harris explained that the parallel cluster randomized controlled trials were carried out among 85,000 total residents from two sites in Nicaragua and Mexico,[9] and the study included double randomization, interventions, and impact measurements. She said that the primary outcomes were incidence (antidengue antibodies in saliva) in children 3 to 9 years of age, entomological indices, and self-reported recent dengue cases. She reported that, for the primary outcomes across both countries, they found a 29.5 percent decrease in the serological indicators, a 24.7 percent decrease in self-reported cases, and decreases between 35.1 percent and 51.7 percent for entomological indices (see Figure 5-4). She reported that secondary analyses found a 25 percent protective factor from the intervention. It also found that use of the larvicide temephos in water storage containers actually increased the risk of dengue. They surmised that the ministry of health may

---

[9] The two sites were the urban city of Managua, Nicaragua, which has a tradition of community organization, and three coastal regions of Guerrero, Mexico, which includes the Acapulco urban area and the rural areas of Costa Grande and Costa Chica.

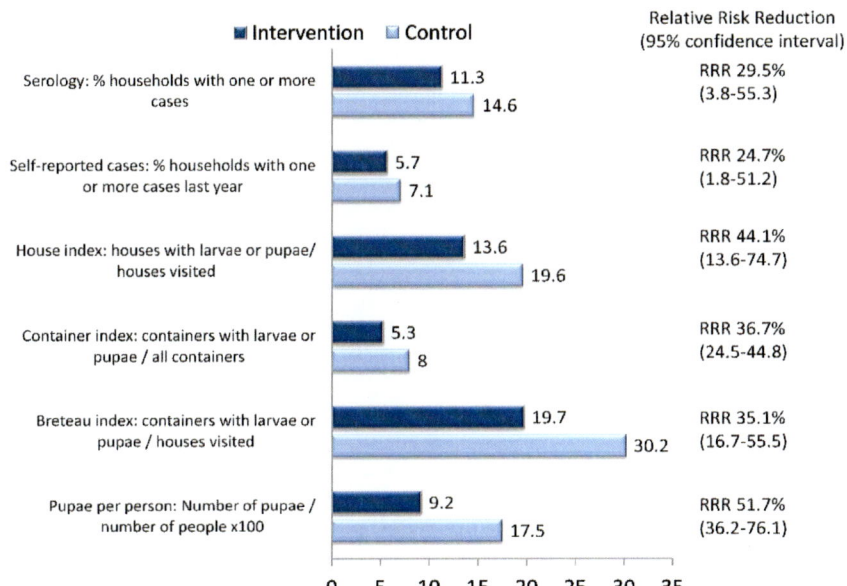

FIGURE 5-4 Primary outcomes of cluster randomized controlled trial Camino Verde, a community involvement intervention across two sites in Nicaragua and Mexico.
NOTE: RRR = relative risk reduction.
SOURCES: Harris presentation, December 13, 2017; data from Andersson et al., 2015.

use temephos in households with notified dengue cases, she added, but the same increase in risk was found in households that had no reported dengue cases. She reported that the same results—decrease in risk with intervention and increase in risk with use of temephos—were obtained over 7 years of the observational pilot study. Social mobilization has been an added value of the intervention, according to Harris. She said that communities have mobilized to have sewer lines placed, for example, by counting the number of barrels and presenting that to the mayor's office. This in turn provides a platform to mobilize on other issues such as domestic and sexual violence, she added. Dengue is the banner, Harris said, but the ability to mobilize on other issues is actually more important to the communities.

DengueChat for Real-Time Capture and Use of Data

Harris reported that they have taken the concepts learned from the Camino Verde and added a technological tool that captures real-time data:

The DengueChat Web– and cell phone–based platform. She explained that the cell phone–based system enables community participation as well as data generation by facilitating the reporting and eliminating of mosquito breeding sites, and community mapping. It also facilitates data capturing through household surveys, socioeconomic status data, and real-time, crowd-sourced community entomology, she said. The accompanying Web-based system allows for communication and dialogue as well as providing specific information for households to use, she added.

A DengueChat user finds a breeding site, takes photographs to document it, then receives points for eliminating it, Harris explained, with the advantage that the information is mapped and the breeding site is destroyed at the same time. This has given rise to "dengue warriors" who compete against each other both individually and as communities, she said. A DengueChat pilot study was carried out in late 2014 and early 2015, she said (Coloma et al., 2016). She reported that pre- and postintervention larva measurements indicate that the brigades kept the work going after the intervention ended in barrios that received the intervention, and those barrios had much lower larva levels than the reference communities almost 2 years later. DengueChat pilots and programs are ongoing in Brazil, Mexico, Nicaragua, and Paraguay, she said.

Harris highlighted the role of community action and community participation in research and data generation in moving toward sustainable models of community engagement. She said there is tension between vertical and horizontal programs, noting that programs have to be housed somewhere, but they also have to be horizontal to work well. She also suggested that a challenge moving forward will be to find ways for ministries of health and community organizations to work together with health, municipal services, and community organizations operating within a complex, integrated, and intersectoral model. She concluded by maintaining that evidence-based actions and policies are critical to first making programs successful and then being able to bring them to scale.

DISCUSSION

David Relman, professor of medicine at Stanford University, asked Harris about what local community members understood to be the measurable goal that was relevant to their daily lives from her studies. Harris responded that they communicated to community members that dengue was a problem that could be addressed by cutting the life cycle of mosquitos to prevent the virus from being transmitted. She said they explained that a person can be infected with dengue but not be sick and that when there is another infection it can be worse. Harris said that showing people that their own children had dengue infection was powerful and catalyzed community engagement in understanding the mosquito life cycle and why breeding sites need to be eliminated—many community members became citizen scientists through this process, she said. They also solicited testimonials, she added, such as, "My son had dengue hemorrhagic fever and it was very frightening," or "My brother died of it." Harris emphasized that the communities were engaged because the community collected evidence including larvae and pupae in their own homes, as well as test results indicating whether their children had the infection, even if the children were not sick.

Relman followed up by asking if there were general features of those measurable goals that made them particularly compelling for the local populations. Harris replied that since the large-scale trial has finished, the focus has shifted to entomological evidence that does not require serological analysis in a laboratory. More broadly, she said, the focus should be on tangible evidence that people can measure and use to track progress, but this will vary according to what the intervention is targeting. In that context, Lantagne noted that WASH does not have a similarly tangible goal as the elimination of mosquito breeding sites. She said that treating water reduces the number of diarrhea cases in children under 5 years of age by half, but fewer diarrhea cases is not as strong of a driver in WASH as the fear of cholera. Much of the desired behavior change has been seen around cholera outbreaks and epidemics.

Lantagne also mentioned that when behavior research was conducted, common responses to the reason for behavior change included statements that denote aspirational thinking, such as, "I have a good family, I am going to take care of my children, and I want to provide my guests something nice." She also provided an example from Haiti where people like the tap on the safe water storage container because it makes them look as if they have flowing water in the household. However, she noted that the triggers for aspiration-motivated behavior change will vary for different cultures and interventions. On the other hand, she remarked that there is ethical debate in sanitation over using the disgust reaction as motivation.

Agarwal described his efforts to work with a population of about 300,000 people spread across 54 slums, collecting qualitative community-level outcome indicators that can be measured over time to demonstrate progress. For example, he said a community would be assigned a color-coded dot (green, yellow, or red) that indicates the proportion of households that have toilets in a community or the proportion of households that have an adequate water supply for general use. Agarwal said they use similar outcome indicators to measure the work of community groups as well as for governance purposes (for example, to indicate whether the community was exercising its power and entitlements to demand assistance from the government). These are important measurements that can propel immediate action.

Peter Daszak, president of EcoHealth Alliance, wondered how the presenters have dealt with governments that oppose or disenfranchise some populations that are purposefully pushed to live in slums or low-income settings due to ethnicity, political ideology, class, or immigration status. Agarwal responded that his program initially faced opposition from the government for using the phrase "illegal slum" instead of "listed slum," for example. He said that after extensive meetings over time, they were able to help shift some of the thinking at the government level, which has now become part of the National Urban Health Mission. Lantagne remarked that, in her experience, governments are resistant to reporting to WHO diseases such as cholera, regardless of the population affected. Such tensions move back and forth, she noted, and suggested that efforts need to align within that to understand where the balance is. She continued that this type of imbalance is evident in some refugee camps in places like Kenya, where the governments provide refugees with the minimum amount of water for human survival and the refugees provide the government with host-country status and the consequent funding and political will.

Nabarro asked why the types of approaches described by the presenters are not happening everywhere. He hypothesized that one issue is the need to change the narrative and suggested that it should be a collective responsibility in this work to help build a methodology that centrally includes shifting the narrative, which applies to health and beyond. For example, he suggested shifting the language from the concept of telling people top-down about how to change behaviors to the concept of helping to enable and empower people. He posited that this amounts to a move from instructing to engaging, from engaging to encouraging participation, and from encouraging participation to stimulating ownership and local management. He suggested that programs might explicitly include a focus on trust building with local authorities as well as conveying that a given program is not a tool for local authorities to manipulate. Nabarro also suggested that, for an approach to be widely adopted, it is important to have a clear methodology that can be taught and learned. Lantagne added that this type of shift is reflected in the language that is becoming more widespread in emergency response now: rather than the cost-prohibitive mass provision of water filters, for example, the approach to an emergency has shifted to finding an inflection point or nudge, such as how to get chlorine into the country to treat the water trucks. She noted that the term *compliance* implies that "those poor people didn't comply with me and treat their water," and said that it is essential to move toward understanding the community and its potential nudges. Harris said that in both Mexico and Nicaragua they carefully mapped out the so-called SEPA strategy, which identifies and illustrates how to approach the critical pieces in each country. In terms of changing the narrative, she said that in vector control there is an openness to new strategies to supplant those that are not working, as well as an openness to having the community be part of the story. She noted that governments tend to be vested in standard approaches because, even if they are not effective, they demonstrate that something is being done to deal with an epidemic. Another problem, according to Harris, is the heavy financial investment of industry in those standard approaches, which she said gives rise to larger meta-political and economic issues. Lindsay suggested that these interventions can also be seen as development, which contributes to improved health. Agarwal added that, in his experience, it is important to work collaboratively with communities and local authorities; to use the appropriate polite, nonconfrontational language; and to make materials and meetings specific and focused.

Edward You, supervisory special agent in the Federal Bureau of Investigation's Weapons of Mass Destruction Directorate, asked Harris if they measured potential financial or other impacts from decrease in disease. Harris said that some of the data captured include how many days someone was out because of their sick child or themselves. She added that the motivation behind new barrios taking part in the large trial came from a cost study and focus groups that showed the amount of money spent on mosquito control, which triggered looking for effective alternatives.

Umair Shah, executive director of the National Association of County & City Health Officials, asked about engaging the marginalized to imbue resilience and positivity in a bidirectional way toward a common understanding of health. He also asked about how to translate some of the work from global settings to domestic settings in the United States. Harris replied that they have created a platform similar to DengueChat, called ZikaChat, which includes a mosquito control component as well as tools and information about how to deal with Zika and pregnancy. In the San Francisco Bay Area, she said, there are efforts to engage communities in mosquito abatement, and she reported that there has been receptivity on the local domestic side for incorporating some elements from global health that make sense in this domestic environment. Lantagne said that work done in decentralized WASH in emergencies in developing countries has been brought back to the United States when there is an emergency, such as the necessary use of household water filters in Flint, Michigan, caused by infrastructure problems. She noted that some types of interventions not previously distributed in the United States are now being used for short-term interventions after hurricanes, for example.

In the larger sense, Lantagne remarked, people are beginning to question how long the U.S. water and sewer infrastructure can be maintained in order to meet the regulations for new chemicals each year while continuing to provide 150 gallons per person per day of quality drinking water to every individual in the United States. She suggested that if practices such as watering lawns with drinking-quality water are not changed, then there may be a secondary sanitary revolution to contend with, especially with the advent of more emergencies related to climate change and infrastructure.

Albert Ko, professor and chair of the Department of Epidemiology of Microbial Diseases at the Yale School of Public Health, asked whether latrines are a viable long-term solution for urban slum populations, especially in megacities. Lantagne replied that latrines do not make sense in urban slums because of the issue of space for sludge disposal. There are also concerns about their viability in rural areas, partially because children tend to be afraid of latrines, and their feces end up on the ground. Furthermore, she noted that, even though latrines isolate waste from the environment, the people handling the waste have increased risk of disease and transmission. She suggested that the narrative should be changed away from latrines in general and toward other options, such as providing people toilets and collection or providing centralized places to defecate.

Ko remarked that in situations of poverty or when high negative health externalities are present, it is difficult to think of approaches that do not include subsidies or conditional cash transfers in the implementation pathway of trying to increase coverage. Lantagne replied that emergency response and development are both moving in the direction of conditional or unconditional cash transfers, because giving cash is efficient and it stimulates the local economy.

Emily Gurley, associate scientist in the Department of Epidemiology at the Johns Hopkins Bloomberg School of Public Health, asked whether technology could help facilitate communities in collecting their own data and in monitoring their own exposure and health status, noting that some communities are already monitoring their own air pollution. Lantagne said that there is a significant move toward funding new technologies for rapid water testing, because the current limitation is that most of the ways to test this require either a culture or polymerase chain reaction, which both take time.

As moderator of the session, Corburn synthesized some of the concepts he gleaned from the presentations. Questions to address moving forward, he said, include how to move from research into action, policy, and intervention as well as what to do, for whom, how to do it, and how to assess what is working. He noted that the presentations emphasized the role of community members as experts, not just in consultation for research but as active contributors to identifying problems, collecting and analyzing data, moving toward solutions, and evaluating progress. Communities and cities are complex systems rather than monocultures, he reflected, and suggested that integrating local expertise and knowledge could help to better understand risks and effective interventions. Corburn said that slums should not be approached in the context of only one exposure, behavior, or risk at a time; he suggested making the eco-bio-social-cultural interaction explicit in this work and considering how people and places co-constitute risk exposure. He remarked that the problems at hand are too complex and challenging to be addressed by a priori models and solutions; he added that community engagement can be integrated with building robust monitoring, tracking, and data feedback systems to allow for continuous adjustment. Finally, Corburn suggested that linkages between policy and local, urban, and community-scale projects appear to be a critical piece in moving to health equity.

6

Bridging Drivers and Interventions to Scale Up Successful Practices

The final session of the workshop focused on bridging drivers and interventions to scale up successful practices in urban and slum health. The session was moderated by Mary Wilson, clinical professor of epidemiology and biostatistics at the University of California, San Francisco. During the session, the workshop organizers requested that forum members, speakers, and attendees break into three groups to explore three different assigned themes related to the promotion of health in urban environments. Each group was moderated by a workshop speaker or a member of the Forum on Microbial Threats.

Participants in group 1 were asked to consider integrated strategies that promote health and health equity on the national and local levels in low-income urban settings. This group was moderated by Jason Corburn, director of the Institute of Urban and Regional Development and professor of public health and of city and regional planning at the University of California, Berkeley. In group 2, participants were charged with discussing scaling up successful practices from research to practice in local communities. Group 2 was moderated by Thomas Scott, distinguished professor of entomology and nematology at the University of California, Davis. Participants in group 3 focused on the business case for investing in health-promoting urban environments and the link to the Sustainable Development Goals (SDGs). This group was moderated by Christopher Dye, director of strategy, policy, and information at the Office of the Director-General, World Health Organization (WHO).

This chapter summarizes potential priorities for research and action that emerged from the breakout groups and reflections on possible next steps by some workshop participants during the final synthesis discussion of the workshop. The ideas from each group should not be construed as collective conclusions or recommendations, and do not necessarily represent the views of all workshop participants, the Forum members, or the National Academies.

PROMOTING HEALTH AND HEALTH EQUITY IN LOW-INCOME URBAN SETTINGS

Jason Corburn, director of the Institute of Urban and Regional Development and professor of public health and of city and regional planning at the University of California, Berkeley, reported for the group that focused on integrated strategies that promote health and health equity in low-income urban settings. He said that individuals in the group framed their discussion along five areas related to urban health equity:

1. Community engagement
2. Building a local workforce
3. Gathering data
4. Moving research into policy
5. Prioritizing slum health in existing institutions

Community Engagement

According to Corburn, the group discussed the value of working toward a rich and robust definition of what community means, which may not be adequately captured by local or international institutional definitions. He said that community members are valuable experts, idea generators, and investigators who could contribute in meaningful ways to health promotion efforts throughout the process, not just after the fact, as they are the ones who often understand the community's problems as well as its needs. Through this ongoing engagement, the interventions and solutions may be more tailored, equitable, accessible, and context specific.

The group discussed models from other disciplines that may offer useful examples of community engagement, such as community-based participatory research in sociology and anthropology, said Corburn. He added that meaningful engagement with the urban poor could be bolstered by efforts to explicitly recognize and openly discuss structural drivers, including racism and spatial segregation, which contribute to health inequities, such as lack of access to health and other essential services. He said the group also discussed the strategy of engaging with place-based characteristics that influence people's opportunities, such as social, cultural, and environmental issues.

Building a Local Workforce

Corburn reported that the group explored ways that community engagement strategies can build a local workforce. He suggested that there is an opportunity for the urban poor to benefit economically through community engagement and through the research and practice of slum upgrading if researchers are intentional about building local capacity and leadership. He explained that this model of both science and action with long-term engagement has the potential to create employment opportunities, which could be beneficial for organizations that are already active on the ground or for groups that are already disenfranchised from the economy (such as the youth). He said the group also discussed the role of community health workers and how to create a trajectory for community health workers to better integrate into the professional health worker pipeline. Corburn suggested that efforts toward building a local workforce could play a part in local-level economic development to address issues such as urban poverty.

Gathering Data

Participants spoke about the need for more data on slums as well as better, disaggregated data, said Corburn. Individuals in the group examined the possibility of developing an urban, slum-specific national data system. The data could be collected through the census, he said, or through urban slum surveillance providing longitudinal data, as was seen in examples from India and Kenya in workshop presentations. This information could uncover the realities of slum health and be leveraged to create more accountability and urgency by decision makers to act and improve slum conditions. As some governments take responsibility for certain large slums but not always for other slums and informal settlements, Corburn said the group discussed broadening the definition of slums to be more inclusive of unlisted slums in India, for example, perhaps through the mandate of WHO or another international organization. He noted that WHO has pushed for urban air pollution data across thousands of cities, for example, and wondered whether something similar might be achieved through local support and local capacity building around urban and slum health issues. Corburn suggested that longitudinal data could be helpful for tracking what is happening in slums. He noted that the one constant in cities and slums is change, suggesting that change could be seen as an opportunity to track and measure what is happening in places around the world as well as who is benefiting and who is not by using "natural experiments."

Moving Research into Policy

The fourth point discussed by the group, said Corburn, was how to bridge the gap between research and existing institutional decision making and policy. He said that individuals in the group pointed out that researchers in the medical and biomedical fields may not clearly understand that policies in cities can act as opportunities or barriers to health improvements. To that end, he said that participants in the group suggested training researchers to better understand those opportunities and barriers and helping them build the skills to engage with policy makers on nonhealth issues, such as transportation, housing, and economic development. The group also discussed, according to Corburn, whether WHO or other international organizations could use their influence to take on a greater role in slum health by developing an urban and slum health program.

Prioritizing Slum Health in Existing Institutions

The final point considered by his group, said Corburn, was potential opportunities available within existing institutions to incorporate work on urban and slum health. For example, the group discussed that academic institutions might refocus training around urban and slum health, because few global health programs offer explicit training in this field in a holistic, interdisciplinary, and organized fashion, he said. Similarly, according to Corburn, the group discussed whether sponsors and funders might consider rerouting funding and resources based on real areas of need as identified through community outreach and improved data. It can be difficult to obtain funding for work on the types of urban and slum health activities discussed during the workshop, he said, because funding tends to be more narrowly focused on specific diseases or exposure. Developing new means of engagement with the different foundations might help to address this, he added. Participants in the group generated a list of disciplines that could be part of an interdisciplinary approach to urban and slum health to bring a range of perspectives into research, practice, and pedagogy. This list includes anthropology, medicine, epidemiology, public health, sociology, economics, civil and environmental engineering, urban planning, geography, microbiology, data science, demography, modeling, policy making, education and knowledge translation, law, ethics, media and communication, and community mobilization.

Jonna Mazet, executive director of the One Health Institute at the University of California, Davis, underscored the issue of institutional encouragement to help sponsors and governments to be more cognizant that this type of One Health or interdisciplinary approach requires support. As Corburn mentioned earlier, Mazet emphasized that financing still tends to go toward single diseases and issues, which has the effect of accidentally discouraging interdisciplinary participation, especially around community engagement. She suggested that this might be addressed by encouraging—or even requiring—funding proposals to include this type of interdisciplinary approach.

SCALING UP SUCCESSFUL PRACTICES: LEARNING FROM LOCAL COMMUNITIES

Thomas Scott, distinguished professor of entomology and nematology at the University of California, Davis, reported for the group tasked with exploring opportunities to scale up successful practices by learning from local communities. The group framed their discussion using four questions:

1. What are the key components for successfully scaling up public programs in local and/or urban environments?
2. How can and should public health scale-up be integrated with other development programs?
3. How do we create a translational pathway from basic science to operational research to health policy, implementation, and impact in low-income urban settings?
4. Does one size fit all, or do we have to tailor intervention scale-up to each city?

Scaling Up Public Health Programs in Local Urban Environments

Scott said the group deliberated about potential components for successfully scaling up public health programs in local urban environments. Sustainability was seen as an important component to many members of the group, which could be reinforced if the intervention contributes not only to its intended purpose but also to other positive community outcomes, explained Scott. For example, as illustrated in the workshop presentation earlier in the day (see Chapter 5) by Eva Harris, professor of infectious disease and vaccinology and director of the Center for Global Public Health at the University of California, Berkeley, a group of youth involved in eliminating mosquito larvae in Nicaragua also applied their combined capacity to address community violence, so a short-term intervention transitioned to fill a long-term community need. Community participation and sufficient coverage to achieve desired outcomes were also discussed as valuable factors with respect to scaling up programs, he said. In the context of outcomes, he added, individual group members suggested setting measurable, meaningful outcomes that are not limited to public health, as well as working toward consensus on goals across sectors involved in urban structure and functional development.

Scott said that other components of successful scale-up were highlighted by the group, including creating an implementation plan, involving multidisciplinary expertise, adapting to the local culture and circumstances, and promoting equity with a long-term view. He also noted that, while there have been successful public health programs that could be scaled up, they were often driven by charismatic individuals, and when such individuals leave, the programs dissolve. To avoid this, Scott reported, the group discussed the potential value of establishing an institutional home to ensure continuity and having key champions train and counsel successors moving into these leadership roles.

Scaling Up and Integrating Public Health with Other Development Programs

Regarding the potential to scale up and integrate public health with other development programs, Scott said, the group discussed the aim of reaching consensus across sectors involved with the structure and function of urban environments. The group examined the potential need to identify and engage leaders who have the will and power to implement these programs, while being cognizant of political and private interests that might help or hinder program scale-up and implementation. The group also discussed developing a plan for scale-up and integration that encompasses management, governance, finance, and leadership. Scott said the group explored the issue of large infrastructural improvements versus disease-specific responses, with the assumption that both long- and short-term solutions are needed. Group members also discussed how ensuring security in the community can be a motivating factor to implement these solutions, he said, as well as the value of coordination among partners and increasing cross-talk and awareness about the benefits of urban development.

Creating a Translational Pathway from Science to Policy

The group considered strategies for creating a translational pathway from basic science to operational research to health policy implementation, said Scott, with a focus on the potential effect of that pathway in low-income urban settings. Participants in the group highlighted the potential role of using a science-driven, evidence-based approach to inform policy, he said, and discussed the types of studies in urban development that would lead to improving public health as well as the role of policy beyond implementation and monitoring. He noted that the translational pathway is not necessarily sequential; that is, policy can be developed concurrently with operational science and implementation. According to Scott, individuals in the group spoke about the benefit of a pipeline for multidisciplinary development, because the current disease-specific approach can be fragmented. The group discussed that institutional support for investing in core sites, such as urban slums, could serve as an incubator for developing an evidence base, said Scott. That base could be bolstered, he said, by integrating data from sites that already have infrastructure in place.

Tailoring Location-Specific Intervention Scale-Up

According to Scott, the group addressed the topic of tailoring the scale-up of interventions for specific cities because one size does not fit all. Participants in the group highlighted the potential usefulness of having a framework for the method and protocol for design and implementation of an intervention, while leaving flexibility for each community to fill in the details that fit their needs and goals, explained Scott. He also noted that the group discussed the value for implementation science to support this type of large-scale change, which could include translatable protocols, a cohort of young professionals with appropriate training and expertise, and sustainable partnerships and collaborations. Scott noted that there are lessons to be learned from existing successful public health efforts, including HIV in Africa, polio eradication, and climate change communication. The group discussed that these lessons could be examined at workshops among multidisciplinary stakeholders to stimulate dialogue and spur an exchange of ideas that has not been facilitated to the fullest extent.

BUILDING THE BUSINESS CASE FOR INVESTING IN HEALTH-PROMOTING URBAN ENVIRONMENTS

The third group examined how to build a business case for investing in health-promoting urban environments. Christopher Dye, director of strategy, policy, and information at the Office of the Director-General, WHO, reported that the group's discussion covered five areas:

1. Conceptualizing a business case for investing in health
2. Inclusion of key players
3. Potential links to the SDGs
4. Distinctiveness of urban environments
5. Potential case studies and evidence base

Conceptualizing a Business Case for Investing in Health

Dye explained that, in this context, building a business case requires defining how to evaluate returns on investment in urban and slum health. He added that the notion of return on investment, for example, is more broadly conceived than it might be in the private sector. Based on the group's discussion, it is not simply about financial investment, he said, but also about social and political investments that cannot always be precisely quantified. The group also discussed that the purpose and audience are important to consider when making each business case, reported Dye. He noted that the outputs of the business case can extend beyond health and well-being to factors that are critical to other stakeholders, such as peace, security, employment, and education. Additionally, some members of the group recognized that even a business case that is strictly financial in terms of its inputs and outputs warrants comprehensive micro- and macro-level economic analyses to evaluate the return on investment beyond those financial terms, said Dye. For example, investments in health can make people more capable for employment or education.

Inclusion of Key Players

The group considered questions about who is developing the business case and for whom, according to Dye. Many of the group members discussed that the community should be fully active in developing the business case, reported Dye, because it is their health that is at stake. The group discussed the possibility of providing the community with veto power on proposed investments from the public or private sector, he said. Other players involved in the business case, Dye added, may include the government; industry; nongovernmental organizations, such as faith-based organizations; and large- and small-scale funders and investors, including local entrepreneurs. The group considered that the research design and evaluation expertise of the academic community can also play a role in developing the business case, said Dye.

Potential Links to the Sustainable Development Goals

The potential contribution of the SDGs to developing a business case was also examined, said Dye. He suggested that the SDG framework could be helpful in that it lays out the potential interactions among its goals and the possibilities for bringing other players into developing the business case. He cautioned that, although the SDGs call for long-term investment in health, the case for actually making those investments will need to be built more specifically and more persuasively while keeping the context and audience in mind. Dye also noted that, in the group's discussion on multisectoral action, many participants recognized that health may not play a dominant role within the broader realm of investment in urban development.

Distinctiveness of Urban Environments

The group discussed the characteristics that make urban environments distinct from other types of environments that may make this business case unique, Dye said. He remarked that by 2050 the majority of the world's population will live in urban areas; he predicted that the people living in towns and cities will influence what happens at the country level. He noted that urban areas tend to be highly active economically with large entrepreneurial communities. The group also discussed that people live at relatively high density, he added, which has implications for the provision of services and infrastructure, some of which could be positive—for example, the volume of people in slums can be an asset for selling increased economies of scale in the water sector. Participants in the group considered that the business case for health in an urban environment might have special features that would not apply in less densely populated rural environments, noted Dye. Urban environments are also characterized by rapid change that gives rise to potential benefits and challenges, including those related to inequities, he said.

Potential Case Studies and Evidence Base

The group explored how amassing a broad range of case studies could be helpful in building an empirical evidence base for establishing best practices, said Dye. This could be used to make the business case for investing in urban and slum health as part of development, he added. Dye referred to the United Nations Human Settlements Programme's (UN-Habitat's) database mentioned in his presentation (see Chapter 2) that includes about 5,000 case studies on developments in the urban environment as a valuable resource. The SDGs can stimulate multisectoral actions, Dye remarked, which have the potential to bring people together through shared finances, combined expertise, and other advantages as well. However, he noted that the health outcomes of multisectoral actions can be hard to discern and measure. He suggested building a better evidence base around the effectiveness of different types of multisectoral actions.

SYNTHESIS AND GENERAL DISCUSSION

The discussion opened with addressing potential ways to build a strong business case that would encourage investments in urban and slum health.

Lonnie King, professor and dean emeritus at The Ohio State University College of Veterinary Medicine, remarked that several years prior, the push toward advancing and adopting corporate social responsibilities in corporations had used language about business cases; he suggested more effectively exploiting that type of language when talking about social responsibility in urban and slum health. Peter Daszak, president of EcoHealth Alliance, noted that in cities where the rich are living and working in such close proximity to the disenfranchised and poor, health represents a connection between them (through disease vectors and transmission) that they might not otherwise have. He suggested leveraging this connection to pitch business cases that will make sense to politicians and decision makers. Daszak also suggested another pitch point for potential business cases: leveraging the connection that wealthier people have with their domestic workers by highlighting the macroeconomic benefit of improving the health of those who are contributing to the country's economy. Albert Ko, professor and chair of the Department of Epidemiology of Microbial Diseases at the Yale School of Public Health, commented that, while the geographical distance may be short between the rich and the poor, there is a great degree of social distance and marginalization. He suggested that the most compelling externality in health is probably violence, but those externalities and root drivers are still poorly understood. Daszak replied that, nonetheless, talking to powerful people in countries where the wealthy are juxtaposed against extreme poverty may drive those in power to do something. Daszak called for acknowledging and confronting policy makers with the relationship between city design and inequities around health care and violence mitigation.

Kent Kester, vice president and head of translational science and biomarkers at Sanofi Pasteur, raised the issue of how to assess the value and generalizability of interventions against the transmission of microbial threats in slums. He suggested harmonizing potential interventions with operational and implementation research components to assess the practical value of proposed interventions. Corburn agreed about the value of fleshing out implementation and evaluation sciences. Scott suggested that measurements should not be limited to public health outcomes. As an example, he questioned whether randomized controlled trials should be considered the gold standard for assessing effectiveness aimed at improving the infrastructure of modern megacities.

Dye said that building an evidence base requires characterizing the quality of the evidence, which can range from anecdotal evidence to randomized controlled trial results. He noted that people who champion randomized control trials around implementation research are probably in the minority, however, and that judgments are most commonly made by people on the ground to make sense of the underlying causes for a program's success or failure. The classification of different levels of evidence is also part of creating a body of relevant case studies, he added, by evaluating a given case study's validity and generalizability. Dye said that some case study databases already exist from UN-Habitat and WHO, for example, although the studies are not all health specific. For guidance about systems for evaluating evidence, Dye suggested looking at WHO's formal classification scheme for developing guidelines for good clinical research practice or the Cochrane systematic reviews, among others. He also suggested collaborating to devise a system for handling more informal types of evidence.

Eric Mintz, team lead for global epidemiology in the Waterborne Diseases Prevention Branch of the U.S. Centers for Disease Control and Prevention, commented that the Global Task Force on Cholera Control released the publication *Ending Cholera—A Global Roadmap to 2030*[1] in October 2017. He suggested that it could be leveraged to improve health in slums and informal settlements in cities, because it proposes to bring large-scale, long-term infrastructure solutions together with the delivery of short-term cholera vaccines in areas that have high incidence or high transmission rates of cholera (which are not necessarily the same spots). Mintz noted that cholera rates are increasing in cities in sub-Saharan Africa because of the growth of informal settlements and periurban areas, where people are vulnerable to waterborne diseases. He added that the road map has identified hot spots in places like Kibera in Nairobi, Kenya, and other large slums and informal settlements where a large cholera epidemic is a potential threat.

David Nabarro, advisor for health and sustainability at 4SD, described his multipart hypothesis of what he defined as a new narrative on how best to contribute to better health of poor urban residents, not only in developing countries but around the world, which is different from the way urban work has conventionally been carried out. The first element, he suggested, is readiness to refashion interventions from the viewpoint of the user and from the viewpoints of the different sectors involved. The second element, he said, is to reform implementation with community ownership and leadership at the center, with statutory bodies facilitating and sometimes nudging when needed to achieve progress. The third element, he continued, is to renew engagement in this work so that instead of slum health being seen as primarily the role of the governments or municipalities, the approach incorporates a range of both private and public actors, such as small-scale entrepreneurs, larger businesses, civil society, faith groups, and scientists. The fourth element, he suggested, is to review financing to focus on leveraging small amounts of resources within local communities to effect change. Nabarro explained that this narrative of building around

---

[1] *Ending Cholera—A Global Roadmap to 2030* is available at www.who.int/cholera/publications/global-roadmap/en (accessed February 10, 2018).

community leadership, horizontal action, and multistakeholder engagement has implications for aspects ranging from the skill mix required from the workforce to development of the business case for investment. He asked the workshop participants if the elements he described are indeed part of a new narrative that is worth pursuing, or if an alternative route should be considered.

Dye responded that it may be the beginnings of a new narrative, although it is not yet sufficiently formed to be considered a new way of doing business in development. He cautioned against taking that step too quickly, which may lead to past mistakes, such as the sudden decision to support structural adjustment influenced by major funding agencies. He further warned that a jump toward a general model of development both in urban areas and more widely should be justified by the evidence. He remarked that it is useful to consider Nabarro's proposed narrative as a hypothesis to be tested for broader generalizability, alongside other ideas at various stages of development. Scott commented that the narrative described by Nabarro may be worth pursuing, but it is unclear how to best proceed with such an approach. Rather than starting from scratch, Scott suggested bringing together important players in the field with a diverse set of expertise and conducting a systematic review of existing data.

Corburn agreed with Nabarro's premises, while emphasizing the need to take a more accelerated approach. Corburn explained that the proposed narrative is not necessarily new, as a corpus of literature exists from community development and participatory practice, for example, which demonstrates the positive effects of this type of framework. To move toward the framework proposed by Nabarro, Corburn suggested that taking an aggressive approach would be better than a slow one because the current crisis of health and inequities in cities demands significant attention. Corburn articulated the "need to build the evidence base by doing, not by just studying," arguing that the evidence base needs to be built quickly through action, such as pilot programs, coupled with evaluating and tracking multiple effects.

Harris remarked that there is evidence to support the approach of "learning by doing" and pushing forward to try bringing some of those approaches to scale, despite the challenges inherent in scaling up and scaling out. She agreed with Corburn that the narrative described by Nabarro is not necessarily a new one, but she noted that it is getting more traction in an increasing number of arenas. Scott cautioned that methods for "learning by doing" need to be done carefully, such as choosing the type of evidence base, to avoid wasting resources and generating unintended consequences for already vulnerable populations. Harris clarified that she is not advocating for "learning by doing" at a global scale, but rather gaining lessons from a pilot stage that may serve as the principles for the next phase. She suggested that certain principles need to be followed, but communities benefit from learning what works at their own level. In that sense, she said, it is possible to have a strong, rigorous methodology that is not one size fits all. Harris added that when there is an evidence base available—from a randomized controlled trial, for example—trying to scale it up beyond the level of a study is an important next step. Scott responded that there is a balance to strike between addressing urgent needs quickly and making informed decisions based on an appropriate evidence base, even though randomized controlled trials are expensive and time consuming.

Dye remarked that the discussion had been focused on top-down initiatives and noted the importance of other types of initiatives that self-propagate within communities and spread quickly. He described the example of M-Pesa, a platform that allows users to make payments using mobile phones. He said that mobile money was unsuccessfully launched by telephone companies in South Africa, but when it spread to Kenya, where bank branches are scarce, people quickly adopted it, reaching community members who they had not imagined were interested in using this platform (Suri and Jack, 2016). He cited this as an example of the general phenomenon of good ideas spreading through communities on their own, without being driven by external panels of experts making decisions about evidence quality. These types of self-propagating innovations could be further examined, Dye suggested.

King observed that communities in poor, rural settings are clever and often have been able to survive and sustain themselves over time through creative means and wondered if there is any work around possibilities for engaging with communities through entrepreneurship to reduce poverty and improve health. Scott responded that it could be a good opportunity to take an existing proof of concept and then implement it with sufficient scale, time, and space to achieve the public health outcome being sought.

Jay Siegel, retired chief biotechnology officer and head of scientific strategy and policy for Johnson & Johnson, raised the issue of big data. He remarked that the city of Chicago has modeled multiple factors, such as the outbreak of foodborne illnesses in relation to the proximity of restaurants and exposed garbage, which increased the efficiency of rodent control efforts (NASEM, 2016). Given the amount of data that he presumes is being collected at various community and health department levels, he asked if there are opportunities to learn more about what works by analyzing data that have already been collected. Corburn replied that there is both inequity and opportunity in big data. He explained that a wealth of data available from various sources have not yet been analyzed in ways that relate those interventions to health or health determinants. He added that ample opportunities exist to increase the available data that are specific both to populations and to places that are either unrecognized, understudied, or not typically captured by government data.

Alex Ezeh, former executive director of the African Population and Health Research Center in Kenya, suggested encouraging countries to identify urban clusters and slums in the 2020 census. He noted that much work in slums is focused on big cities and mega-slums rather than in smaller towns that are becoming slums in their entirety because of a lack of urban planning and provision of services. He predicted that this type of decentralization will pose a challenge going forward because smaller slum dynamics are different from slums in big cities. Ko added that trends in urbanization in developing countries show that much of the growth is in midsize cities rather than megacities and noted that midsize cities experience quantitatively and qualitatively different problems than megacities.

Ko also raised the issues of equity in the interventions chosen among all other options to implement and equity in the implementation of those interventions. In other words, he said, it is the issue of "poor solutions for poor people." He questioned why people in slums are often provided with inferior solutions masked to be innovative when there are, in fact, evidence-based solutions that should be implemented, as sometimes is the case with water, sanitation, and hygiene interventions. Emily Gurley, associate scientist in the Department of Epidemiology at the Johns Hopkins Bloomberg School of Public Health, replied that asking the most marginalized people to do the most for safe water—to treat it at the household level—is an inequity. She said that the root cause of the issue is poor governance that does not support these vulnerable populations, because infrastructure ultimately depends on governance and large projects rather than short-term emergency solutions.

Corburn described Medellín, Colombia, as an example of positive urban transformation—it went from being the most violent city in the world in the early 1990s to no longer placing in the top 100 cities in terms of gun homicides. He explained that this was not achieved through aggressive policing or occupation, but through a complex process of deep investment in infrastructure and public spaces. Corburn attributed the success in Medellín to a combination of innovation in leadership, planning for transformation, and strong community engagement. They also used a strategy called participatory budgeting that allowed residents to prioritize certain aspects, he added, as well as the innovative use of existing technology, such as ski lifts and escalators for public transportation.

Corburn said that another strategy employed with significant health impact was called the "ethics of aesthetics," placing beautiful buildings, museums, and libraries in the poorest neighborhoods. He suggested that there are lessons to be learned from the equity of the interventions that transformed Medellín. Espinal suggested building upon existing best practices from places like Medellín and from *favelas* in Brazil that have been completely modernized in terms of security and continuing to highlight the importance of health in all policies. Nabarro emphasized that the people collectively involved in setting the standards for health must avoid cheap and substandard solutions for poor people's ill health, if only for the reason that poor people often have much less room than rich people to maneuver if things go wrong. He suggested that the designs of interventions for poor communities are usually based on less robust and resilient approaches than the interventions designed for rich communities.

David Relman, professor of medicine at Stanford University, asked whether there are strategies for homogenizing the urban landscape in slums (other than reducing density) that might address the problem of disease transmission. Corburn replied that, if by homogenizing Relman is referring to living standards and conditions, then there has been evidence of bad planning as the result of trying to homogenize. He said that the city of Brasilia in Brazil was well planned by modern standards, but the workers who migrated to build the city created their own informal settlement on the periphery, which became the interesting part of the city. People on the edges of city planning tend to talk about how planning relates to health and disease, he added, but most people tend to like cities because they are dynamic, fun, social places with opportunities for different types of expression. Corburn expressed concern about the term *homogenization* because the richness of urbanization is its diversity. He suggested that intersectoral efforts should aim to balance efforts to address disease and exposure scenarios while simultaneously maintaining the diversity, richness, beauty, and cultures that make cities healthy at their core.

Ezeh reiterated that, in many cases, the health solutions brought to bear for poor, vulnerable populations are poor policies that end up damaging more than healing. The necessary solutions and interventions are often simple and affordable, he added, but they require working jointly with the communities. His biggest concern is "the best being the enemy of the good," he said. While it would be ideal to wait until the most scientifically proven intervention can be implemented, he explained, a basic intervention available today could also be implemented. Ezeh emphasized that if communities were listened to and collaborated with using the resources currently available, it would make a significant difference in the lives of many people living in slums today.

CLOSING REMARKS

To close the workshop, James Hughes, professor of medicine and public health at the Emory University Rollins School of Public Health, outlined a set of needs that were suggested throughout the workshop and which resonated from his perspective:

- Continued emphasis on the relevance of the SDGs;
- Strengthening the evidence base;
- Including health in all policies;
- Engaging communities, local experts, and policy makers in planning;
- Promoting the empowerment of women;
- Placing emphasis on collaboration across disciplines and sectors, in line with the One Health approach;
- Promoting equity;
- Moving beyond disease-specific solutions; and
- Thinking broadly about return on investment in health.

Relman reflected on the framing of issues during this workshop and noted that there seemed to be more consideration of the intersection of theory and reality, of the "end game," and of taking action and measuring effects than in previous forum workshops. He underscored Ezeh's remark about preventing the perfect from being an enemy of the good and encouraged the group to continue working on improved measures and interventions, while continuing to implement available and effective interventions. Relman suggested focusing on the science of implementation for known interventions, while also exploring other aspects of basic science, such as microbiology and molecular biology and engineering, which might contribute to decision making. Relman concluded by emphasizing the importance of striking a balance in both considerations of more experimental studies such as those that may help better understand ecological dispersal across slum environmental circumstances and the urgency of scaling up demonstrable interventions as presented throughout the workshop.

Appendix A

References

Achee, N. L., F. Gould, T. A. Perkins, R. C. Reiner, Jr., A. C. Morrison, S. A. Ritchie, D. J. Gubler, R. Teyssou, and T. W. Scott. 2015. A critical assessment of vector control for dengue prevention. *PLoS Neglected Tropical Diseases* 9:e0003655.

Alirol, E., L. Getaz, B. Stoll, F. Chappuis, and L. Loutan. 2011. Urbanisation and infectious diseases in a globalised world. *The Lancet Infectious Diseases* 11(2):131–141.

Andersson, N., E. Nava-Aguilera, J. Arosteguí, A. Morales, H. Suazo-Laguna, J. Legorreta, C. Hernandez-Alvarez, I. Fernandez Salas, S. Paredes-Solís, A. Balmaseda, A. Juan Cortés-Guzmán, R. Serrano de Los Santos, J. Coloma, R. J. Ledogar, and E. Harris. 2015. Evidence based community mobilization for dengue prevention in Nicaragua and Mexico (Camino Verde, the green way): Cluster randomized controlled trial. *BMJ* 351:h3267.

Andrews, J. R., C. Morrow, R. P. Walensky, and R. Wood. 2014. Integrating social contact and environmental data in evaluating tuberculosis transmission in a South African township. *The Journal of Infectious Diseases* 210(4):597–603.

APHRC (African Population Health Resource Center). 2002. *Population and health dynamics in Nairobi's informal settlements: Report of the Nairobi Slums Survey (NCSS) 2000.* Nairobi, Kenya: African Population and Health Research Center.

Azman, A. S., J. Lessler, S. M. Satter, M. V. McKay, A. Khan, D. Ahmed, and E. S. Gurley. 2015. Tracking cholera through surveillance of oral rehydration solution sales at pharmacies: Insights from urban Bangladesh. *PLoS Neglected Tropical Diseases* 9(12):e0004230.

Bairoch, P., and G. Goertz. 1986. Factors of urbanisation in the nineteenth century developed countries: A descriptive and econometric analysis. *Urban Studies* 23(4):285–305.

Barden-O'Fallon, J., M. A. Barry, P. Brodish, and J. Hazerjian. 2015. Rapid assessment of Ebola related implications for reproductive, maternal, newborn and child health service delivery and utilization in Guinea. *PLoS Currents* 7.

Beguy, D., P. Elung'ata, B. Mberu, C. Oduor, M. Wamukoya, B. Nganyi, and A. Ezeh. 2015. Health and demographic surveillance system profile: The Nairobi Urban Health and Demographic Surveillance System (NUHDSS). *International Journal of Epidemiology* 44(2):462–471.

Belser, J. A., A. M. Eckert, T. M. Tumpey, and T. R. Maines. 2016. Complexities in ferret influenza virus pathogenesis and transmission models. *Microbiology and Molecular Biology Reviews* 80(3):733–744.

Bi, Q., A. S. Azman, S. M. Satter, A. I. Khan, D. Ahmed, A. A. Riaj, E. S. Gurley, and J. Lessler. 2016. Micro-scale spatial clustering of cholera risk factors in urban Bangladesh. *PLoS Neglected Tropical Diseases* 10(2):e0004400.

Câmara, E. J., J. C. Braga, L. S. Alves-Silva, G. F. Câmara, and A. A. da Silva Lopes. 2002. Comparison of an intravenous pulse of methylprednisolone versus oral corticosteroid in severe acute rheumatic carditis: A randomized clinical trial. *Cardiology in the Young* 12(2):119–124.

Câmara, E. J., C. Neubauer, G. F. Câmara, and A. A. Lopes. 2004. Mechanisms of mitral valvar insufficiency in children and adolescents with severe rheumatic heart disease: An echocardiographic study with clinical and epidemiological correlations. *Cardiology of the Young* 14(5):527–532.

Casanovas-Massana, A., F. Costa, I. N. Riediger, M. Cunha, D. de Oliveira, D. C. Mota, E. Sousa, V. A. Querino, N. Nery, Jr., M. G. Reis, E. A. Wunder, Jr., P. J. Diggle, and A. I. Ko. 2018. Spatial and temporal dynamics of pathogenic *Leptospira* in surface waters from the urban slum environment. *Water Research* 130:176–184.

Castro, M., L. Sánchez, D. Pérez Chacón, N. Carbonell, P. Lefèvre, V. Vanlerberghe, and P. Van der Stuyft. 2012. A community empowerment strategy embedded in a routine dengue vector control programme: A cluster randomised controlled trial. *Transactions of the Royal Society of Tropical Medicine and Hygiene* 106(5):315–321.

CHP (Centre for Health Protection). 2007. *A review of community-associated methicillin-resistant* Staphylococcal aureus *(CA-MRSA) cases in Hong Kong*. https://www.chp.gov.hk/files/pdf/a_review_of_community-associated_methicillin_resistant_staphylococcal_aureus_ca-mrsa_cases_in_hong_kong_r.pdf (accessed March 12, 2018).

Cifuentes, S. G., J. Trostle, G. Trueba, M. Milbrath, M. E. Baldeon, J. Coloma, and J. N. Eisenberg. 2013. Transition in the cause of fever from malaria to dengue, northwestern Ecuador, 1990–2011. *Emerging Infectious Diseases* 19(10):1642–1645.

Cisse, M., M. S. Diallo, C. T. Tidiane, C. Kpamou, J. Dimitri, E. Dortenzio, and J. D. Ndawinz. 2015. *Impact of the Ebola outbreak on the quality of care of people living with HIV taking antiretroviral treatment at Donka National Hospital in Conakry, Guinea*. Abstract. Paper presented at the Proceedings of the Conference on Retroviruses and Opportunistic Infections, Seattle, WA.

Coloma, J., H. Suazo, E. Harris, and J. Holston. 2016. Dengue chat: A novel web and cellphone application promotes community-based mosquito vector control. *Annals of Global Health* 82(3):451.

Cornwall, W. 2016. A plague of rats. *Science* 352(6288):912–915.

Costa, F., E. A. Wunder, D. De Oliveira, V. Bisht, G. Rodrigues, M. G. Reis, A. I. Ko, M. Begon, and J. E. Childs. 2015. Patterns in *Leptospira* shedding in Norway rats (*Rattus norvegicus*) from Brazilian slum communities at high risk of disease transmission. *PLoS Neglected Tropical Diseases* 9(6):e0003819.

Dick, E. C., L. C. Jennings, K. A. Mink, C. D. Wartgow, and S. L. Inhorn. 1987. Aerosol transmission of rhinovirus colds. *The Journal of Infectious Diseases* 156(3):442–448.

Dye, C. 2008. Health and urban living. *Science* 319(5864):766–769.

Dye, C., B. Bourdin Trunz, K. Lonnroth, G. Roglic, and B. G. Williams. 2011. Nutrition, diabetes, and tuberculosis in the epidemiological transition. *PLoS ONE* 6(6):e21161.

Elston, J. W., A. J. Moosa, F. Moses, G. Walker, N. Dotta, R. J. Waldman, and J. Wright. 2016. Impact of the Ebola outbreak on health systems and population health in Sierra Leone. *Journal of Public Health (Oxford)* 38(4):673–678.

Erlanger, T. E., J. Keiser, and J. Utzinger. 2008. Effect of dengue vector control interventions on entomological parameters in developing countries: A systematic review and meta-analysis. *Medical and Veterinary Entomology* 22(3):203–221.

Ezeh, A., O. Oyebode, D. Satterthwaite, Y. F. Chen, R. Ndugwa, J. Sartori, B. Mberu, G. J. Melendez-Torres, T. Haregu, S. I. Watson, W. Caiaffa, A. Capon, and R. J. Lilford. 2017. The history, geography, and sociology of slums and the health problems of people who live in slums. *The Lancet* 389(10068):547–558.

Gao, X., J. Wei, B. J. Cowling, and Y. Li. 2016. Potential impact of a ventilation intervention for influenza in the context of a dense indoor contact network in Hong Kong. *Science of the Total Environment* 569–570:373–381.

Gates, B. 2014. *The deadliest animal in the world.* https://www.gatesnotes.com/Health/MostLethal-Animal-Mosquito-Week (accessed March 12, 2018).

Government of Hong Kong. 2017. *Labour force characteristics.* http://www.censtatd.gov.hk/hkstat/sub/gender/labour_force (accessed March 12, 2018).

Government of Kenya. 2004. *Kenya demographic and health survey 2003.* Nairobi, Kenya: Government of Kenya.

Griggs, D. J., M. Nilsson, A. Stevance, and D. McCollum. 2017. *A guide to SDG interactions: From science to implementation.* Paris, France: International Council for Science.

Gurley, E. S., M. J. Hossain, R. C. Paul, H. M. Sazzad, M. S. Islam, S. Parveen, L. I. Faruque, M. Husain, K. Ara, Y. Jahan, M. Rahman, and S. P. Luby. 2014. Outbreak of hepatitis E in urban Bangladesh resulting in maternal and perinatal mortality. *Clinical Infectious Diseases* 59(5):658–665.

Gürtler, R. E., and Z. E. Yadon. 2015. Eco-bio-social research on community-based approaches for Chagas disease vector control in Latin America. *Transactions of the Royal Society of Tropical Medicine and Hygiene* 109(2):91–98.

Hacker, K. P., A. Minter, M. Begon, P. J. Diggle, S. Serrano, M. G. Reis, J. E. Childs, A. I. Ko, and F. Costa. 2016. A comparative assessment of track plates to quantify fine scale variations in the relative abundance of Norway rats in urban slums. *Urban Ecosystems* 19(2):561–575.

Heintze, C., M. Velasco Garrido, and A. Kroeger. 2007. What do community-based dengue control programmes achieve? A systematic review of published evaluations. *Transactions of the Royal Society of Tropical Medicine and Hygiene* 101(4):317–325.

Herfst, S., E. J. Schrauwen, M. Linster, S. Chutinimitkul, E. de Wit, V. J. Munster, E. M. Sorrell, T. M. Bestebroer, D. F. Burke, D. J. Smith, G. F. Rimmelzwaan, A. D. Osterhaus, and R. A. Fouchier. 2012. Airborne transmission of influenza A/H5N1 virus between ferrets. *Science* 336(6088):1534–1541.

Hermans, S., C. R. Horsburgh, Jr., and R. Wood. 2015. A century of tuberculosis epidemiology in the northern and southern hemisphere: The differential impact of control interventions. *PLoS ONE* 10(8):e0135179.

Issarow, C. M., N. Mulder, and R. Wood. 2015. Modelling the risk of airborne infectious disease using exhaled air. *Journal of Theoretical Biology* 372:100–106.

Kirking, H. L., J. Cortes, S. Burrer, A. J. Hall, N. J. Cohen, H. Lipman, C. Kim, E. R. Daly, and D. B. Fishbein. 2010. Likely transmission of norovirus on an airplane, October 2008. *Clinical Infectious Diseases* 50(9):1216–1221.

Ko, A. I., M. Galvao Reis, C. M. Ribeiro Dourado, W. D. Johnson, Jr., and L. W. Riley. 1999. Urban epidemic of severe leptospirosis in Brazil, Salvador leptospirosis study group. *The Lancet* 354(9181):820–825.

Kraemer, M. U., M. E. Sinka, K. A. Duda, A. Q. Mylne, F. M. Shearer, C. M. Barker, C. G. Moore, R. G. Carvalho, G. E. Coelho, W. Van Bortel, G. Hendrickx, F. Schaffner, I. R. Elyazar, H. J. Teng, O. J. Brady, J. P. Messina, D. M. Pigott, T. W. Scott, D. L. Smith, G. R. Wint, N. Golding, and S. I. Hay. 2015. The global distribution of the arbovirus vectors *Aedes aegypti* and *Ae. albopictus*. *eLife* 4:e08347.

Kuruvilla, S., J. Schweitzer, D. Bishai, S. Chowdhury, D. Caramani, L. Frost, R. Cortez, B. Daelmans, A. de Francisco, T. Adam, R. Cohen, Y. N. Alfonso, J. Franz-Vasdeki, S. Saadat, B. A. Pratt, B. Eugster, S. Bandali, P. Venkatachalam, R. Hinton, J. Murray, S. Arscott-Mills, H. Axelson, B. Maliqi, I. Sarker, R. Lakshminarayanan, T. Jacobs, S. Jack, E. Mason, A. Ghaffar, N. Mays, C. Presern, and F. Bustreo for the Success Factors for Women's and Children's Health study groups. 2014. Success factors for reducing maternal and child mortality. *Bulletin of the World Health Organization* 92(7):533B–544B.

Lei, H., Y. Li, S. Xiao, X. Yang, C. Lin, S. L. Norris, D. Wei, Z. Hu, and S. Ji. 2017. Logistic growth of a surface contamination network and its role in disease spread. *Scientific Reports* 7(1):14826.

Leuenberger, D., J. Hebelamou, S. Strahm, N. De Rekeneire, E. Balestre, G. Wandeler, and F. Dabis for the IeDEA (International epidemiological Databases to Evaluate AIDS) West Africa Study Group. 2015. Impact of the Ebola epidemic on general and HIV care in Macenta, Forest Guinea, 2014. *AIDS (London, England)* 29(14):1883–1887.

Li, Y., I. T. S. Yu, P. Xu, J. H. W. Lee, T. W. Wong, P. L. Ooi, and A. C. Sleigh. 2004. Predicting super spreading events during the 2003 severe acute respiratory syndrome epidemics in Hong Kong and Singapore. *American Journal of Epidemiology* 160(8):719–728.

Li, Y., X. Huang, I. T. S. Yu, T. W. Wong, and H. Qian. 2005. Role of air distribution in SARS transmission during the largest nosocomial outbreak in Hong Kong. *Indoor Air* 15(2):83–95.

Lilford, R. J., O. Oyebode, D. Satterthwaite, G. J. Melendez-Torres, Y. F. Chen, B. Mberu, S. I. Watson, J. Sartori, R. Ndugwa, W. Caiaffa, T. Haregu, A. Capon, R. Saith, and A. Ezeh. 2017. Improving the health and welfare of people who live in slums. *The Lancet* 389(10068):559–570.

Liu, L., Y. Li, P. V. Nielsen, J. Wei, and R. L. Jensen. 2017. Short-range airborne transmission of expiratory droplets between two people. *Indoor Air* 27(2):452–462.

Marlow, M. A., E. L. Maciel, C. M. Sales, T. Gomes, R. E. Snyder, R. P. Daumas, and L. W. Riley. 2015. Tuberculosis DALY-gap: Spatial and quantitative comparison of disease burden across urban slum and non-slum census tracts. *Journal of Urban Health* 92(4):622–634.

Matossian, M. K. 1997. *Shaping world history: Breakthroughs in ecology, technology, science, and politics.* Armonk, NY: M.E. Sharpe.

McBride, A. J., D. A. Athanazio, M. G. Reis, and A. I. Ko. 2005. Leptospirosis. *Current Opinion in Infectious Diseases* 18(5):376–386.

Morrison, A. C., E. Zielinski-Gutierrez, T. W. Scott, and R. Rosenberg. 2008. Defining the challenges and proposing new solutions for *Aedes aegypti*-borne disease prevention. *PLoS Medicine* 5:362–366.

Morse, B., K. A. Grepin, R. A. Blair, and L. Tsai. 2016. Patterns of demand for non-Ebola health services during and after the Ebola outbreak: Panel survey evidence from Monrovia, Liberia. *BMJ Global Health* 1(1):e000007.

NASEM (National Academies of Sciences, Engineering, and Medicine). 2016. *Big data and analytics for infectious disease research, operations, and policy: Proceedings of a workshop.* Washington, DC: The National Academies Press.

NSSO (National Sample Survey Organisation). 2010. Some characteristics of urban slums, 2008–09: NSS 65th round, July 2008–June 2009. New Delhi, India: National Sample Survey Office, National Statistical Organisation, Ministry of Statistics and Programme Implementation, Government of India.
Pang, X., P. Yang, S. Li, L. Zhang, L. Tian, Y. Li, B. Liu, Y. Zhang, B. Liu, R. Huang, X. Li, and Q. Wang. 2011. Pandemic (H1N1) 2009 among quarantined close contacts, Beijing, People's Republic of China. *Emerging Infectious Diseases* 17(10):1824–1830.
Parpia, A. S., M. L. Ndeffo-Mbah, N. S. Wenzel, and A. P. Galvani. 2016. Effects of response to 2014–2015 Ebola outbreak on deaths from malaria, HIV/AIDS, and tuberculosis, West Africa. *Emerging Infectious Diseases* 22(3):433–441.
Patrick, M., M. Steenland, A. Dismer, J. Pierre-Louis, J. L. Murphy, A. Kahler, B. Mull, M. D. Etheart, E. Rossignol, J. Boncy, V. Hill, and T. Handzel. 2017. Assessment of drinking water sold from private-sector kiosks in post-earthquake Port-au-Prince, Haiti. *The American Journal of Tropical Medicine and Hygiene* 97(4 Suppl):84–91.
Patterson, B., C. D. Morrow, D. Kohls, C. Deignan, S. Ginsburg, and R. Wood. 2017. Mapping sites of high TB transmission risk: Integrating the shared air and social behaviour of TB cases and adolescents in a South African township. *Science of the Total Environment* 583:97–103.
Perry, H., M. Morrow, S. Borger, J. Weiss, M. Decoster, T. Davis, and P. Ernst. 2015. Care groups I: An innovative community-based strategy for improving maternal, neonatal, and child health in resource-constrained settings. *Global Health: Science and Practice* 3(3):358–369.
Plowright, R. K., C. R. Parrish, H. McCallum, P. J. Hudson, A. I. Ko, A. L. Graham, and J. O. Lloyd-Smith. 2017. Pathways to zoonotic spillover. *Nature Reviews Microbiology* 15(8):502–510.
Pravettoni, R., and UNEP/GRID-Arendal. 2011. *Slum population in urban Africa.* http://www.grida.no/resources/8194 (accessed March 12, 2018).
Reis, R. B., G. S. Ribeiro, R. D. M. Felzemburgh, F. S. Santana, S. Mohr, A. X. T. O. Melendez, A. Queiroz, A. C. Santos, R. R. Ravines, W. S. Tassinari, M. S. Carvalho, M. G. Reis, and A. I. Ko. 2008. Impact of environment and social gradient on *Leptospira* infection in urban slums. *PLoS Neglected Tropical Diseases* 2(4):e228.
Richardson, E. T., C. D. Morrow, D. B. Kalil, S. Ginsberg, L. G. Bekker, and R. Wood. 2014. Shared air: A renewed focus on ventilation for the prevention of tuberculosis transmission. *PLoS ONE* 9(5):e96334.
Santamouris, M., A. Synnefa, M. Asssimakopoulos, I. Livada, K. Pavlou, M. Papaglastra, N. Gaitani, D. Kolokotsa, and V. D. Assimakopoulos. 2008. Experimental investigation of the air flow and indoor carbon dioxide concentration in classrooms with intermittent natural ventilation. *Energy and Buildings* 40(10):1833–1843.
Sesay, T., O. Denisiuk, K. K. Shringarpure, B. S. Wurie, P. George, M. I. Sesay, and R. Zachariah. 2017. Paediatric care in relation to the 2014–2015 Ebola outbreak and general reporting of deaths in Sierra Leone. *Public Health Action* 7(Suppl 1):S34–S39.
Shuaib, F., R. Gunnala, E. O. Musa, F. J. Mahoney, O. Oguntimehin, P. M. Nguku, S. B. Nyanti, N. Knight, N. S. Gwarzo, O. Idigbe, A. Nasidi, and J. F. Vertefeuille. 2014. Ebola virus disease outbreak—Nigeria, July–September 2014. *Morbidity and Mortality Weekly Report.* https://www.cdc.gov/mmwr/preview/mmwrhtml/mm6339a5.htm (accessed March 12, 2018).
Sikder, M., U. Daraz, D. Lantagne, and R. Saltori. 2018. Water, sanitation, and hygiene access in southern Syria: Analysis of survey data and recommendations for responses. *Conflict and Health* 12:17.
Simpson, J. V. A. 1924. A report on the ventilation of schools. *The Journal of Hygiene* 22(2):164–174.

Sommerfeld, J., and A. Kroeger. 2012. Eco-bio-social research on dengue in Asia: A multi-country study on ecosystem and community-based approaches for the control of dengue vectors in urban and peri-urban Asia. *PATH* 106(8):428–435.

Steer, A. C., I. Law, L. Matatolu, B. W. Beall, and J. R. Carapetis. 2009. Global *emm* type distribution of group A streptococci: Systematic review and implications for vaccine development. *The Lancet Infectious Diseases* 9(10):611–616.

Suri, T., and W. Jack. 2016. The long-run poverty and gender impacts of mobile money. *Science* 354(6317):1288.

Tartof, S. Y., J. N. Reis, A. N. Andrade, R. T. Ramos, M. G. Reis, and L. W. Riley. 2010. Factors associated with group A *Streptococcus emm* type diversification in a large urban setting in Brazil: A cross-sectional study. *BMC Infectious Diseases* 10(1):327.

UN DESA (United Nations Department of Economic and Social Affairs). 2015. *World urbanization prospects: The 2014 revision.* New York: United Nations.

UN-Habitat (United Nations Human Settlements Programme). 2003. *Global report on human settlements 2003: The challenge of slums.* Nairobi, Kenya: United Nations Human Settlements Programme.

UN-Habitat. 2006. *The state of the world's cities report 2006/2007: The Millennium Development Goals and urban sustainability.* Nairobi, Kenya: United Nations Human Settlements Programme.

UN-Habitat. 2016a. *Slum almanac 2015-2016: Tracking improvements in the lives of slum dwellers.* Nairobi, Kenya: United Nations Human Settlements Programme.

UN-Habitat. 2016b. *The new urban agenda.* Nairobi, Kenya: United Nations Human Settlements Programme.

UN-Habitat. 2017. *Distinguishing slum from non-slum areas to identify occupants' issues.* Nairobi, Kenya: United Nations Human Settlements Programme.

Vanlerberghe, V., M. E. Toledo, M. Rodriguez, D. Gomez, A. Baly, J. R. Benitez, and P. Van der Stuyft. 2009. Community involvement in dengue vector control: Cluster randomised trial. *The BMJ* 338:b1959.

Verma, G. D. 2002. *Slumming India: A chronicle of slums and their saviours.* New Delhi, India: Penguin Books India.

Vos, T., R. M. Barber, B. Bell, A. Bertozzi-Villa, S. Biryukov, I. Bolliger, F. Charlson, A. Davis, L. Degenhardt, D. Dicker, L. Duan, H. Erskine, V. L. Feigin, A. J. Ferrari, et al. 2015. Global, regional, and national incidence, prevalence, and years lived with disability for 301 acute and chronic diseases and injuries in 188 countries, 1990-2013: A systematic analysis for the global burden of disease study 2013. *The Lancet* 386(9995):743–800.

Walker, P. G., M. T. White, J. T. Griffin, A. Reynolds, N. M. Ferguson, and A. C. Ghani. 2015. Malaria morbidity and mortality in Ebola-affected countries caused by decreased health care capacity, and the potential effect of mitigation strategies: A modelling analysis. *The Lancet Infectious Diseases* 15(7):825–832.

Wei, J., and Y. Li. 2016. Airborne spread of infectious agents in the indoor environment. *American Journal of Infection Control* 44(9 Suppl):S102–S108.

Wells, W. F. 1955. *Airborne contagion and air hygiene: An ecological study of droplet infections.* Cambridge, MA: Harvard University Press.

Wesolowski, A., N. Eagle, A. Tatem, D. Smith, A. Noor, R. W. Snow, and C. O Buckee. 2012. Quantifying the impact of human mobility on malaria. *Science* 338(6104):267–270.

WHO (World Health Organization). 2004. *Global strategic framework for integrated vector management.* Geneva, Switzerland: World Health Organization.

WHO. 2005. *The current evidence for the burden of group A streptococcal diseases.* Geneva, Switzerland: World Health Organization.

WHO. 2013. *Health in all policies: Framework for country action.* Geneva, Switzerland: World Health Organization.

WHO. 2014. *Liberia: Ebola treatment centre sets a new pace.* http://www.who.int/features/2014/liberia-ebola-island-clinic/en (accessed March 12, 2018).
WHO. 2015. *Health worker Ebola infections in Guinea, Liberia, and Sierra Leone: A preliminary report 21 May 2015.* Geneva, Switzerland: World Health Organization.
WHO. 2016. *Global tuberculosis report 2016.* Geneva, Switzerland: World Health Organization.
WHO. 2017a. *Global vector control response 2017-2030.* Geneva, Switzerland: World Health Organization. http://www.who.int/vector-control/publications/global-control-response/en (accessed March 12, 2018).
WHO. 2017b. *Health in the SDG era.* Geneva, Switzerland: World Health Organization.
WHO. 2017c. *Progress on drinking water, sanitation and hygiene.* Geneva, Switzerland: World Health Organization.
WHO and World Bank. 2017. *Tracking universal health coverage: 2017 global monitoring report.* Washington, DC: World Bank Group.
Wilder-Smith, A., D. J. Gubler, S. C. Weaver, T. P. Monath, D. Heymann, and T. W. Scott. 2017. Epidemic arboviral diseases: priorities for research and public health. *The Lancet Infectious Diseases* 17:e101–e106.
Wilner, L., E. Wells, M. Ritter, J. M. Casimir, K. Chui, and D. Lantagne. 2017. Sustained use in a relief-to-recovery household water chlorination program in Haiti: Comparing external evaluation findings with internal supervisor and community health worker monitoring data. *Journal of Water Sanitation and Hygiene for Development* 7(1):56–66.
Wood, R., H. Liang, H. Wu, K. Middelkoop, T. Oni, M. X. Rangaka, R. J. Wilkinson, L. G. Bekker, and S. D. Lawn. 2010. Changing prevalence of tuberculosis infection with increasing age in high-burden townships in South Africa. *International Journal of Tuberculosis and Lung Disease* 14(4):406–412.
Wood, R., C. Morrow, S. Ginsberg, E. Piccoli, D. Kalil, A. Sassi, R. P. Walensky, and J. R. Andrews. 2014. Quantification of shared air: A social and environmental determinant of airborne disease transmission. *PLoS ONE* 9(9):e106622.
Xie, X., Y. Li, A. T. Chwang, P. L. Ho, and W. H. Seto. 2007. How far droplets can move in indoor environments—revisiting the Wells evaporation-falling curve. *Indoor Air* 17(3):211–225.
Yates, T. M., E. Armitage, L. V. Lehmann, A. J. Branz, and D. S. Lantagne. 2015. Effectiveness of chlorine dispensers in emergencies: Case study results from Haiti, Sierra Leone, Democratic Republic of Congo, and Senegal. *Environmental Science & Technology* 49(8):5115–5122.
Zhang, L., and Y. Li. 2012. Dispersion of coughed droplets in a fully-occupied high-speed rail cabin. *Building and Environment* 47:58–66.

Appendix B

Workshop Statement of Task

An ad hoc committee under the auspices of the National Academies of Sciences, Engineering, and Medicine will plan a 1.5-day public workshop that will examine new transmission pathways of microbes in the urban built environment that affect human health. This workshop will feature invited presentations and discussions on the following topics:

- The current state of science of the formation, function, and interaction of microbial communities in the urban built environment that affect human health;
- Specific urban built environment characteristics, spatial heterogeneity, and land-use patterns, as well as social and behavioral factors (host and vector movement) that may alter vector distribution, and increase or facilitate transmission of infectious diseases;
- Critical opportunities, challenges, and knowledge gaps relevant to translating research findings into practical application of shaping urban environments that prevent and mitigate infectious disease outbreaks;
- Innovative strategies, interventions, and policies for creating sustainable and health-promoting urban built environments that consider structural and socioeconomic determinants of diseases;
- Obtaining valid and reliable data to monitor and evaluate implementation and progress of programs and policies; and
- Collaboration and coordination mechanisms among various stakeholders and across sectors in urban planning, public policy, public

health, animal health, environmental health, microbiology, and social and behavioral sciences.

Workshop speakers and discussants will contribute perspectives from government, academia, and the private and nonprofit sectors. The committee will plan and organize the workshop, select and invite speakers and discussants, and moderate the discussions. A proceedings of the presentations and discussions at the workshop will be prepared by designated rapporteurs in accordance with institutional guidelines.

Appendix C

Workshop Agenda

TUESDAY, DECEMBER 12, 2017

1:00 pm ET	Opening Remarks
David Relman, Chair of the Forum on Microbial Threats

Current Challenges and Opportunities for the Prevention and Control of Infectious Diseases in an Increasingly Urban and Interconnected World

Global Perspective:
Christopher Dye, World Health Organization

Local Perspective:
Alex Ezeh, African Population and Health Research Center, Kenya

Workshop Overview and Goals
James Hughes, Workshop Co-Chair
Mary Wilson, Workshop Co-Chair

Session I: Social, Physical, Environmental, and Political Drivers of Infectious Disease Transmission in the Urban Built Environment

Part A: Current State of Science and Knowledge Gaps in an Evolving Landscape
Maria Gloria Dominguez-Bello, *Moderator*

2:00 pm   The Influence of Cities, Urban Environments, and Informal Settlements on Population Health and Microbial Communities
Lee W. Riley, University of California, Berkeley

Understanding Mechanisms and Implications of Human Exposure to Microbes in Urban Buildings: Research Gaps, Opportunities, and Barriers
Yuguo Li, University of Hong Kong

Migration and Movement: Pathways of Pathogens Within, Into, and Out of Urban Centers
David L. Smith, University of Washington

2:45 pm   Discussion

3:30 pm   Break

Part B: Translating Conceptual Models into Practice
Marcos Espinal, *Moderator*

3:45 pm   The Impact of the West Africa Ebola Virus Disease Outbreak on the Epidemiology of Other Infectious Diseases
Frank Mahoney, International Federation of Red Cross and Red Crescent Societies

Water-Borne Diseases in Dhaka, Bangladesh
Emily Gurley, Johns Hopkins Bloomberg School of Public Health

Emerging Vector-Borne and Zoonotic Diseases in the Urban Landscape: Zika and Leptospirosis in Brazilian Slum Settlements
Albert Ko, Yale School of Public Health

	Tuberculosis Transmission in South Africa **Robin Wood,** University of Cape Town
4:45 pm	Discussion
5:25 pm	Wrap Up **Mary Wilson,** Workshop Co-Chair
5:30 pm	Adjourn
5:35 pm	Reception

WEDNESDAY, DECEMBER 13, 2017

8:30 am ET	Welcome **James Hughes,** Workshop Co-Chair
8:35 am	Global Efforts for Leveraging the Sustainable Development Goals and Promoting Healthy Lives (remote presentation) **Steve Lindsay,** Durham University, England

Session II: Effective Interventions and Policies—Achieving Sustainable and Health-Promoting Urban Built Environments
Jason Corburn, *Moderator*

8:55 am	Building an Investment Case for Slum Upgrading and Health-Promoting Urban Environments **Siddharth Agarwal,** Urban Health Resource Centre, India
	Physical and Engineering Interventions Fit for Context: A Focus on Water, Sanitation, and Hygiene **Daniele Lantagne,** Tufts University
	Engaging Communities from Surveillance to Policy **Eva Harris,** University of California, Berkeley
9:45 am	Discussion
10:30 am	Break

Session III: Exploring Research Gaps to Bridge Drivers and Interventions and Scaling Up Successful Practices

10:45 am	Introduction to Session **Eric Mintz,** U.S. Centers for Disease Control and Prevention
10:55 am	(mobilize to breakout room)
11:00 am	Breakout Session
12:30 pm	Lunch
1:30 pm	Breakout group reports **Mary Wilson,** *Moderator* Group 1: Integrated Strategies That Promote Health and Health Equity on the National and Local Levels in Low-Income Urban Settings **Jason Corburn,** University of California, Berkeley Group 2: Scaling Up Successful Practices—From Research to Practice in Local Communities **Thomas Scott,** University of California, Davis Group 3: The Business Case for Investing in Health-Promoting Urban Environments and the Link to the Sustainable Development Goals **Christopher Dye,** World Health Organization
2:00 pm	Synthesis and General Discussion **Mary Wilson,** *Moderator*
3:15 pm	Closing Remarks **James Hughes,** Workshop Co-Chair **Mary Wilson,** Workshop Co-Chair **David Relman,** Chair of the Forum on Microbial Threats
3:30 pm	Adjourn

Appendix D

Biographical Sketches of Workshop Speakers and Moderators

Siddharth Agarwal, M.B.B.S., is a physician who has worked in research and programming in public health, nutrition, maternal and newborn health, community empowerment, urban health planning, and policy support to national and state governments and global public health policy advocacy. He has been working for the cause of well-being, nutrition, and health of disadvantaged populations for 30 years. He is the director of Urban Health Resource Centre (UHRC), a nonprofit organization that works for the health, nutrition, and well-being of 500,000 disadvantaged urban dwellers through demonstration programs in partnership with slum communities and government departments, and it also engages in research, policy support, and advocacy. UHRC played a key role in stakeholder consultations, meetings, and study tours, and consolidating lessons from programs over 6 years for the government of India's National Urban Health Mission that mandates reaching out to all listed and unlisted slums and vulnerable settlements. He has collaborated nationally and internationally with researchers of U.S. and UK universities and institutions on several projects dealing with urban well-being, health, and sustainable development. He teaches public health from a multidisciplinary perspective and is adjunct faculty at the Johns Hopkins Bloomberg School of Public Health and in the Department of Global Health at The George Washington University. He has served as guest faculty at the University of California, Berkeley; TERI University; Institut d'Études Politiques Sciences Po, Paris; Coady International Institute STFX–Canada; Touro College, New York; University of Leeds, United Kingdom; Delhi University, IIT–Kanpur; and Indian Institute of Public Health, Delhi. He has been guiding in-country and overseas Ph.D.

and master's students for the past several years. He has been a member of several government of India committees, a member of several international committees and panels, and an advisor to the World Health Organization (South East Asia Regional Office and Kobe Centre, Japan), United Nations Human Settlement Program, United Nations Population Fund, and United Nations Children's Fund, United Nations University, and the International Society for Urban Health on different aspects of vulnerability, disparities, health care, public health, community health, nutrition, urban health, well-being, policy, practice, and sustainable development. He is the past president of the International Society of Urban Health (2010–2011) and was an executive board member from 2008 to 2014. He is a member of editorial boards and review panels of several international journals and has been a reviewer for The Wellcome Trust, United Kingdom. He has had more than 100 articles, research papers, book chapters, and reports published in Indian and international journals, books, and newspapers. His interviews have been published by governmental and nongovernmental periodicals and newspapers and by international agencies. He is a recipient of an AXA Outlook Award, a nomination-based award of AXA Research Fund, Paris, and the Rotary Vocational Service Award for his services toward the betterment of the underprivileged in 2015. He delivered the Professor Shakuntala Memorial Oration at his alma mater, Lala Lajpat Rai Memorial Medical College, Meerut, at the start of the Medical College's Golden Jubilee year activities in 2016.

Jason Corburn, Ph.D., M.C.P., is the director of the Institute of Urban and Regional Development and a professor in the Department of City and Regional Planning and the School of Public Health at the University of California, Berkeley. His research focuses on environmental justice and climate change in cities, the links between urban planning and public health, and inclusive community development for informal settlements in cities in Africa, Asia, and Latin America. He is a research and evaluation advisor for the World Health Organization, the International Council of Science, and numerous local and national governments. Dr. Corburn has conducted research projects on the health equity impacts of new urban governance strategies in San Francisco and Richmond; sanitation, food security, and community development projects in Nairobi's informal settlements; and community planning, poverty reduction, and infectious disease in Rio de Janeiro and Salvador, Brazil. Dr. Corburn has received numerous awards, including the United Nations Association Global Citizenship Award, the Paul Davidoff Best Book Award, the Health Policy Investigator Award from the Robert Wood Johnson Foundation, and the Environmental Leadership Program Fellowship.

Maria Gloria Dominguez-Bello, Ph.D., received her undergraduate degree in 1983 from Simon Bolivar University, her master's degree in 1987 (animal nutrition), and her Ph.D. in 1990 (microbiology) from the University of Aberdeen, Scotland. In 1993, she was a European Union Marie Curie postdoctoral fellow in the United Kingdom and France. She developed her scientific career to full professor at the Venezuelan Institute of Scientific Research, where she worked for 14 years, and at the University of Puerto Rico, where she worked for 11 years. Since 2012 she has been an associate professor of medicine at the New York University School of Medicine. She is a fellow of the American Academy of Microbiology and of the Infectious Diseases Society of America, and has served as a board member of *Livestock Science*, *Microbial Ecology*, *Frontiers in Microbiology*, *Microbes and Infection*, *mBio*, and *Scientific Reports*. Her lab integrates data from genomics/metagenomics, microbiology, ecology, physiology, and anthropology to address broad questions about microbe–host interaction, including development of the infant microbiota, effect of the Western lifestyle, and microbiota restoration.

Christopher Dye, FRS, FMedSci, is the director of strategy, policy, and information in the Office of the Director-General at the World Health Organization (WHO). Dr. Dye began professional life as an ecologist in the United Kingdom, having graduated from the University of York (B.A., biology) and the University of Oxford (D.Phil., zoology). After developing an interest in infectious diseases at Imperial College London, he moved to the London School of Hygiene & Tropical Medicine to bring his research closer to public health. He was head of the school's Vector Biology and Epidemiology Unit until 1996, carrying out research on leishmaniasis, malaria, rabies, and other infectious and zoonotic diseases in Africa, Asia, and South America. In 1996, he joined WHO, where he has developed methods for using national surveillance and survey data to study the large-scale dynamics and control of tuberculosis, malaria, Ebola, Zika, and other communicable diseases. As director of strategy, he now serves as science advisor to the director-general and other senior staff, oversees the production and dissemination of health information via the WHO press and libraries, and coordinates WHO's sustainable development network. From 2006 to 2009, he was also professor of physics (and other biological sciences) at Gresham College, and 35th in a lineage of professors that have been giving public lectures in the City of London since 1597. He is a fellow of The Royal Society (the UK National Academy of Sciences) and of the UK Academy of Medical Sciences. He is a visiting professor of zoology at the University of Oxford and a member of the Board of Reviewing Editors for *Science*.

Marcos A. Espinal, M.D., Dr.P.H., M.P.H., is the director of the Department of Communicable Diseases and Health Analysis at the Pan American Health Organization (PAHO), Regional Office of the World Health Organization (WHO) for the Americas. Dr. Espinal, a national of the Dominican Republic, holds a medical degree from the Universidad Autónoma de Santo Domingo, Dominican Republic (1985). He has an M.P.H. (1990) and a Dr.P.H. (1995) from the University of California, Berkeley, School of Public Health. His work experience includes positions in the Ministry of Health of the Dominican Republic and the National Center for Research on Maternal and Child Health; the New York City Public Health Department; and WHO, where he worked for 13 years. Before joining PAHO, Dr. Espinal served as the executive secretary of the WHO Stop TB Partnership, a global movement aiming to eliminate tuberculosis as a public health problem. Dr. Espinal has published more than 100 peer-reviewed publications in the field of communicable diseases. He is a recipient of the Scientific Prize of the International Union against Tuberculosis and Lung Diseases; the Walter and Elise A. Hass International Award by the University of California, Berkeley, for a distinguished record of service in international health; and the Princess Chichibu Memorial Tuberculosis Global Award by the Japan Anti-Tuberculosis Association.

Alex Ezeh, Ph.D., stepped down as the executive director of the African Population and Health Research Center (APHRC) on September 30, 2017, after 17 years. As the founding executive director, Dr. Ezeh guided APHRC to become one of Africa's foremost regional research centers addressing population, health, education, and development issues. He initiated and directed the Consortium for Advanced Research Training in Africa, an initiative to strengthen doctoral training and the retention of academics at African universities. He was a member of The Rockefeller Foundation–Lancet Commission on Planetary Health and the Lancet Commission on the Future of Health in Africa. He currently co-chairs the Guttmacher-Lancet Commission on Sexual and Reproductive Health in a post-2015 world. Dr. Ezeh is honorary professor of public health at the University of the Witwatersrand, South Africa, and holds an honorary doctor of science degree from KCA University, Kenya, and a doctorate in demography from the University of Pennsylvania. He serves on the boards of several organizations, including the United Nations University–International Institute for Global Health (Kuala Lumpur), the World Health Organization's Alliance for Health Policy and Systems Research (Geneva), and the International Initiative for Impact Evaluation (3ie).

Emily Gurley, Ph.D., M.P.H., is an associate scientist in the Department of Epidemiology at the Johns Hopkins Bloomberg School of Public Health. She leads multidisciplinary studies on the transmission and prevention of emerging and vaccine preventable diseases, such as Nipah virus, hepatitis E virus, and arboviruses. She has worked in Bangladesh for more than a decade, and her interests include improving the communication and collaboration between field epidemiologists and infectious disease modelers and development of novel surveillance strategies. Her research adopts a One Health approach to the study and prevention of infectious disease, taking into account the ecological context in which disease occurs. Dr. Gurley is the co-director for the Child Health and Mortality Prevention Surveillance site in Bangladesh, which aims to determine the etiology of and prevent child deaths. She also works closely with the U.S. Centers for Disease Control and Prevention's Global Disease Detection program.

Eva Harris, Ph.D., is a professor in the Division of Infectious Diseases in the School of Public Health and the director of the Center for Global Public Health at the University of California, Berkeley. She has developed a multidisciplinary approach to study the molecular virology, pathogenesis, immunology, epidemiology, clinical aspects, and control of dengue, Zika, and chikungunya, the most prevalent mosquito-borne viral diseases in humans. Specifically, her work addresses immune correlates of protection and pathogenesis, viral and host factors that modulate disease severity, and virus replication and evolution using in vitro approaches, animal models, and research involving human populations. This has been possible through a close collaboration with the Ministry of Health in Nicaragua for more than 28 years. Her international work focuses on laboratory-based and epidemiological studies of dengue, chikungunya, Zika, and influenza in endemic Latin American countries, particularly in Nicaragua, where ongoing projects include clinical and biological studies of severe dengue; a pediatric cohort study of dengue, Zika, chikungunya, and influenza transmission in Managua; a household transmission study of Zika; and a recently concluded cluster randomized controlled trial of evidence-based, community-derived interventions for prevention of dengue via control of its mosquito vector. She is also directing a study of Zika in infants and pregnancy in Nicaragua and evaluating a number of Zika diagnostic tests with her team in Nicaragua. In 1997, she received a MacArthur Award for work over the previous 10 years developing programs to build scientific capacity in developing countries to address public health and infectious disease issues. This enabled her to found a nonprofit organization in 1998, Sustainable Sciences Institute (www.sustainablesciences.org), with offices in San Francisco, Nicaragua, and Egypt, to continue and expand this work.

Dr. Harris was named a Pew Scholar for her work on dengue pathogenesis. She received a national recognition award from the Minister of Health of Nicaragua for her contribution to scientific development and was selected as a "Global Leader for Tomorrow" by the World Economic Forum. In 2012, she was elected Councilor of the American Society of Tropical Medicine and Hygiene and received a Global Citizen Award from the United Nations Association. She has published more than 200 peer-reviewed articles, as well as a book on her international scientific work.

Albert Icksang Ko, M.D., an infectious disease physician, is a professor and the chair of the Department of Epidemiology of Microbial Diseases at the Yale School of Public Health and a collaborating researcher at the Oswaldo Cruz Foundation in the Brazilian Ministry of Health. His research centers on the health problems that have emerged as a consequence of rapid urbanization and social inequity. Dr. Ko coordinates a research and training program on urban slum health in Brazil and is conducting prospective studies on rat-borne leptospirosis, dengue, meningitis, and respiratory infections. His research particularly focuses on understanding the transmission dynamics and natural history of leptospirosis, which works as a model for an infectious disease that has emerged in slum environments due to the interaction of climate, urban ecology, and social marginalization. Current research combines multidisciplinary epidemiology, ecology, and translational research-based approaches to identify prevention and control strategies that can be implemented in slum communities. Dr. Ko is also the program director at Yale for the Fogarty Global Health Equity Scholars Program, which provides research training opportunities for U.S. and low- and middle-income country post- and predoctoral fellows at collaborating international sites. Since December 2016, the research and training program in the city of Salvador, Brazil, has mobilized its efforts to investigate the ongoing outbreak of Zika virus infection and microcephaly.

Daniele Lantagne, Ph.D., is an associate professor in civil and environmental engineering at Tufts University. She is a public health engineer (Massachusetts Institute of Technology [MIT], B.S., 1996; M.Eng., 2001; P.E., 2003) who received her Ph.D. in 2011 from the London School of Hygiene & Tropical Medicine. She began working in water, sanitation, and hygiene to reduce the burden of infectious disease while earning her master's degree, and continued working in this field teaching in the Department of Civil and Environmental Engineering at MIT until she joined the U.S. Centers for Disease Control and Prevention in 2003. She completed her postdoctoral work at Harvard's Center for International Development from 2010 to 2012, and joined Tufts University as a professor in 2012. Over the past 16 years, Dr. Lantagne provided technical assistance or conducted research in more than 50 countries in Africa, Asia, and Central and South America in both development and emergency contexts. She has published more than 50 papers on water supply, water treatment, hygiene, and sanitation in developing countries and is a technical advisor to Potters for Peace, FilterPure, and charity: water. Her main research interest is how to reduce the burden of infectious diseases by investigating and evaluating the effectiveness of water and sanitation interventions. She runs an active group completing laboratory, field, and policy research and currently supervises one postdoctoral student and six Ph.D. and undergraduate researchers with funding from agency, government, nongovernmental organization, foundation, and private sources.

Yuguo Li, Ph.D., is a professor and the associate dean (research) of engineering and former head of the Department of Mechanical Engineering at the University of Hong Kong. He studied at Shanghai Jiaotong University, Tsinghua, and KTH Royal Institute of Technology in Stockholm, and was a principal research scientist at the Commonwealth Scientific and Industrial Research Organisation. His main research interests are on built environment engineering (indoor air quality, city climate, and environmental studies of infection). Recently his team received a collaborative research fund from the Hong Kong government to study how microbes are transmitted on the surface network and indoor contact network in a large city. He led the development of 2009 World Health Organization guidelines on natural ventilation. Professor Li currently serves as an associate editor of *Indoor Air*, and he is the president of the International Society of Indoor Air Quality (ISIAQ) Academy of Fellows. He received the John Rydberg Gold Medal from SCANVAC in 2014, an honorary doctor degree from Aalborg University, Denmark, in 2015, and the Inoue Memorial Award from the Society of Heating, Air-conditioning, and Sanitary Engineers, Japan, in 2016. He was elected a fellow of ISIAQ, as well as the American Society of Heating, Refrigerating, and Air-conditioning Engineers; the Hong Kong Institution of Engineers; and the Institution of Mechanical Engineers.

Steve Lindsay, Ph.D., is a public health entomologist with a passion for studying some of the world's most important vector-borne diseases, including malaria, lymphatic filariasis, dengue, and trachoma. He has considerable experience in medical entomology, parasitology, ecology, and clinical epidemiology and solves pure and applied problems in the laboratory and field using a wide range of techniques from DNA fingerprinting and mathematical modeling to methods used by social scientists, epidemiologists, and biologists. His particular interest is in the design of simple tools for malaria control, and he has carried out field studies in Burkina Faso, China,

Ethiopia, Gambia, Kenya, Laos People's Democratic Republic, Tanzania, Thailand, and Uganda over the past 30 years. He has published more than 200 peer-reviewed papers, many in major international journals. He was in one of the leading groups of researchers in the 1980s that demonstrated that insecticide-treated bed nets protected children against malaria. Since then he has helped develop and carry out field trials of topical repellents, larval source management, combinations of long-lasting insecticidal nets and indoor residual spraying, new resistance-busting mosquito nets, and house screening. He is an advocate for integrated vector management and the improvement of housing as a protection against vector-borne diseases. He has an honorary chair in public health entomology at the London School of Hygiene & Tropical Medicine, is a co-chair of the Vector-borne Diseases and the Built Environment work stream of Roll Back Malaria, and is a member of the World Health Organization's Vector Control Advisory Group and Technical Advisory Group for Neglected Tropical Diseases. He is also the co-director of the Building Out Vector-borne diseases in Africa network (BOVA).

Frank Mahoney, M.D., is an infectious disease epidemiologist who is currently working for the Global Immunization Division (GID) at the U.S. Centers for Disease Control and Prevention (CDC). He is a graduate of the University of Texas Medical School in Houston and completed a residency in family medicine at Baylor University. He joined the CDC in 1989 as an Epidemic Intelligence Service officer and has worked on a variety of assignments throughout his career. He is currently seconded by GID to the International Federation of the Red Cross and Red Crescent Societies. In 2014–2015, he was the CDC team lead for Ebola response in Nigeria and Liberia. Prior to the Ebola outbreak, he was the CDC team lead for polio eradication in Nigeria. Between 2007 and 2011, he was head of the CDC office in Indonesia, and prior to that assignment, he worked for 10 years in the Middle East Region, including 4 years at the Eastern Mediterranean Regional Office (EMRO) of the World Health Organization and 6 years with the U.S. Naval Medical Research Unit No. 3 in Cairo. He is a member of the EMRO Technical Advisory Group on Immunization and the author of numerous scientific publications and book chapters. He is a member of the John Snow Society and an adjunct faculty member at the Emory University Rollins School of Public Health.

Eric Mintz, M.D., M.P.H., obtained his medical degree from the State University of New York in 1984, completed an internal medicine residency at Harlem Hospital in 1987, and received a master in public health from Columbia University in 1989. He joined the U.S. Centers for Disease Control and Prevention as an Epidemic Intelligence Service officer that year, where he has since worked on approaches to prevent waterborne and foodborne diseases in the Americas, Africa, and Asia. Dr. Mintz has authored or co-authored more than 170 scientific publications on topics including typhoid and paratyphoid fever, cholera, dysentery, and new technologies to make safe drinking water, safe sanitation, and better hygiene more accessible, affordable, and sustainable in developing countries.

Lee W. Riley, M.D., is a professor and the head of the Division of Infectious Disease and Vaccinology at the School of Public Health, University of California, Berkeley. He is a physician who has been trained in both epidemiology and molecular microbiology. Dr. Riley did his undergraduate studies at Stanford University, where he received a B.A. in philosophy. He went to medical school at the University of California, San Francisco, and completed a residency in internal medicine at Columbia-Presbyterian Hospital in New York. After residency, Dr. Riley joined the Epidemic Intelligence Service at the U.S. Centers for Disease Control and Prevention (CDC), and then became an infectious disease fellow at the Stanford University School of Medicine. After the fellowship, he joined the World Health Organization to work as a project manager for a program called India Biomedical Support Project in New Delhi, India, for 2 years. Dr. Riley became an assistant professor of medicine at the Cornell University Medical College in 1990, and transferred to the University of California, Berkeley, in 1996 as professor of infectious diseases. He currently directs a research training program called Global Health Equity Scholars program, a consortium of four institutions—University of California, Berkeley; Yale University; Stanford University; and Florida International University—which is funded by the National Institutes of Health's Fogarty International Center, designed to provide training for U.S. and lower- and middle-income country postdoctoral fellows and scholars in slum health research. In 2004, Dr. Riley was elected fellow of the American Academy of Microbiology, and in 2014 he was appointed by the U.S. secretary of health and human services to serve as a member of the Board of Scientific Counselors to advise the Office of Infectious Diseases at the CDC. His research work includes tuberculosis, drug-resistant bacterial infections, and infectious diseases of urban slums. He has research collaborations in Bangladesh, Brazil, China, Colombia, India, Japan, and eastern Europe.

Thomas W. Scott, Ph.D., received his Ph.D. in ecology from The Pennsylvania State University, was a postdoctoral fellow in epidemiology at the Yale School of Medicine, and was a faculty member at the University of Maryland before relocating in 1996 to the University of California, Davis, where he is a distinguished professor of epidemiology and prevention of mosquito-transmitted disease. He aims to assess current recommendations for disease prevention, test assumptions in public health policy, and develop innovative, cost-effective, and operationally efficient concepts for prevention of mosquito-borne disease. He has worked in Latin America, Southeast Asia, and Africa, with an emphasis on longitudinal studies of dengue in Peru and Thailand.

David L. Smith, Ph.D., is a professor of global health at the Institute for Health Metrics and Evaluation (IHME) at the University of Washington. Professor Smith studied ecology and evolutionary biology at Princeton University with Professor Simon A. Levin before moving into epidemiology and global health. Professor Smith's scientific research has been on the ecology, epidemiology, and evolution of infectious diseases. He has published extensively on the epidemiology, dynamics, and control of malaria, influenza, cholera, rabies, *Staphylococcus aureus*, and nosocomial pathogens; the evolution of resistance to antibiotics in nosocomial pathogens; the evolution of resistance to antimalarial drugs; malaria elimination and eradication; and the bioeconomics of infectious diseases. Professor Smith was one of the original members of the Malaria Atlas Project, which has published evidence-based global maps of *Plasmodium falciparum* and *P. vivax*. At IHME, he works closely with the geospatial team, and his interests have expanded to include robust policy interventions to reduce all causes of mortality in children under 5 years of age. A key interest has been to develop analytical tools to compare simple and abstract compartment models to exquisitely detailed individual-based models to answer, What kinds of models (or modeling processes) tend to give the most robust policy advice? This research supports the translation of the output of sophisticated Bayesian geostatistical analysis—particularly the estimates of spatial uncertainty—into usable advice about how, where, and when to distribute interventions.

Robin Wood, D.Sc., FRS, is an infectious diseases physician, an emeritus professor of medicine at the University of Cape Town, South Africa, and the director of the Desmond Tutu HIV Centre at the Institute of Infectious Disease and Molecular Medicine. He gained his medical degree at Oxford University and completed his specialist medical training at the University of Cape Town, followed by an infectious disease fellowship at Stanford University. He has published more than 450 scientific articles in the areas of HIV, infectious diseases, and tuberculosis (TB). He currently leads a multidisciplinary research team focusing on the aerobiology of TB transmission.